NIGHT SKY

To Margaret,

All best wishes

from

Laurence.

LAURENCE E. FISHER

© Laurence E. Fisher 2004
NIGHT SKY DREAMING

ISBN 0-9547585-0-1

Published by:
Kite Publications
32 Pykerley Road
Monkseaton
Whitley Bay
NE25 8EW

Design & production co-ordinated by:
The *Better Book* Company Ltd
Havant
Hampshire
PO9 2XH

Printed in England

CHAPTER ONE

She was standing alone, waiting for me. I climbed the steps slowly, catching my breath, watching and afraid to blink. Her dress, the pale blue of a winter sky, was blowing tightly against her, dark hair billowing forwards. I noted the slenderness of her legs, the graceful arc of her back. The flickering sea, which so captivated her attention, swayed and curved in my ears. It had been two days since we first met, and already I missed her badly.

Nan stood with one leg bent behind the other, both elbows resting on the smooth surface of the wall. She leaned forwards. Two pigeons appeared suddenly from the sea below and she jerked upright, surprised, her hands now gliding gently, rhythmically, over the heat of the stone. In the distance, a cathedral dome glinted sharp golden sunbeams.

I began to cross the road and it seemed that Nan knew exactly where I was. She turned quickly, holding her arms straight out from her body, making the shadow of a cross. Nan smiled and it was then that I knew for sure. I rushed up to her, into her embrace, and into our new life.

'It's so good to see you, Harry. I thought you might have got lost.' She spoke hurriedly, a little nervous.

'Couldn't get away from the hospital.' I pressed my face into her hair, breathing in the warm musk perfume. Her arms tightened over my back. 'You've not been waiting long, have you?'

'I finished early, so I thought I'd come down anyway. The sea is so wonderful, I could watch it for hours. But I'm glad you're here now.' She squeezed my shoulders. 'Come on, we're going somewhere different today.'

Our hands found each other, fingers enlacing, as if they had been doing this for years. Nan led me towards the old fort.

'So what have you been up to today, Harry?'

'Just the usual, getting the hospital ready for action. If I never have to grease another bed frame I'll be a happy man.' Her laughter arrived as an explosion of joy. 'You know what it's like. And the smell of carbolic acid. Ugh! It feels like it's burnt into my nostrils, I can't get rid of it.'

'It could be worse, you know. I've been in surgery today, two gall bladders, one appendix. One of the soldiers was really young too, terrified. I felt so sorry for him.'

'No way. He's lucky Nan, to have you looking after him.'

She smiled, her eyes bright, bending close to kiss my cheek. 'You've shaved?'

'Just now. I promised, didn't I? Can't go making a mess of you.'

Kingsway was on our right, the main street, but we ignored this and kept on walking, the uneven stone of the pavement frequently throwing us together. We passed the giant old fort, now manned and armed again, a flood of shadowed apartments and balconies. The dusty air felt scorched, over-brewed. White seabirds spiralled into the sky.

'So where are you taking me, Nan?'

'The Grand Harbour. It's where you would have arrived.'

I shuddered involuntarily at the memory of that voyage. There had been many moments of danger, "adventure" the Captain had called it, which were too close for comfort. It had been my first real taste of war, and I was glad of nursing duties to keep me occupied. It was the first time someone had died in my arms; I'd never forget that.

'What's wrong, Harry?' Nan noticed my changed expression.

'Just remembering getting here. It wasn't good.'

She pulled me to a stop and we kissed, my hands held loose on her back. There was an obvious kindness to Nan, sensitivity, revealed in her eyes. 'It will be better today, I promise,' she said. 'You're with me now.'

Minutes later, we had descended stone steps and sat on rocks overlooking the harbour. 'I wish you could have seen this before, Harry. It was wonderful.'

The Grand Harbour still appeared magnificent. It was huge, as impressive as the city it enclosed, but I now noticed the twisted masts of sunken ships sticking up from beneath the surface of the glass-green water. I hadn't spotted these in the excitement of arrival. Wherever I turned my eyes, ruin and destruction stared back. The harbour entrance was partially blocked from the Italian E-boat attack; across the water Vittoriosa and Senglea looked to be collapsed. Craters and fallen buildings surrounded us, together with broken wooden beams sticking out like amputations. The few roads that remained passable were badly damaged, all others obstructed with massive piles of rubble.

'What happened?' It was the worst hit area I had seen.

'A lot of this was done when *Illustrious* was here, Harry. It was dreadful, and they still didn't manage to sink her. The attacks seemed to go on forever. We could hear them all the time, at the hospital. I couldn't sleep for days, we were so busy. But at least it bound the people together, that's good.'

'It must have been incredible. Absolute hell.' I hoped that the worst of the bombing was now over, although the Major had suggested otherwise.

'It was. This is my home, Harry. I hate to see it like this.'

'I know what you mean. London's been flattened as well.'

'Of course.' She touched my arm. 'Let's talk about other things, can we?'

The words now tumbled from our lips in their haste to escape, and I learned much more about Nan. I was in a hurry to know everything as quickly as possible.

She was christened Antoinette, after one of the Catholic saints, but nobody except close family called her this. And only then when she was in trouble. She was native to the island and, like most of the people, fiercely pro-British. They feared how the Germans or Italians would treat them.

The family remained in Marsaxlokk, on the east coast, and this village had also been under attack. Her father was a fisherman, like his father before him. Her mother ran the house and looked after everybody. Nan told me that she was a fantastic cook. She had one sister, Theresa, who was fourteen years old and a beautiful singer. Her brother, Noel, was a bookworm and played the trumpet. It was his dream to travel the world, she said.

For several months, Nan had worked in the surgical wards in Valletta. She enjoyed nursing, but not during the worst of the attacks; the injuries sustained had been awful, senseless, heartbreaking. She missed living with her family, a peaceful life. Nan smiled often, running long, delicate fingers through her shoulder-length hair while the wind brushed it repeatedly over her face. She wore no make-up, unlike most of the women I had seen in the city. I was glad about this; it could not have made her more beautiful.

Nan explained how she usually avoided the Gut, but had been persuaded to venture out on Saturday evening.

'Before the war, I didn't go out at night. I didn't want to. It was a quiet life, but I adored that. Nothing like you Brits, always drinking like fishes!' She pushed a hand against my chest, laughing. 'Really, I didn't want to do anything more. It was a good life.'

'Well I'm glad you came out! And it was only my second time there, you know, but Dicky said I'd like you.'

'He said the same about you.'

Nan's dress had risen to reveal her knees. When I placed a hand on her leg and she didn't move away, I knew we would make love that night. We sat huddled together, watching the glitter and sparkle of the waves. I wrapped an arm about her shoulders and we kissed again, before returning our attention to the sea. There was nobody else around, the only sound that of water lapping on stone. I felt so relaxed. Already, we were comfortable with silence.

'Quick, Harry.' It was Nan who jumped up, pulling me to my feet. 'We've got to get back to Fountain Street.'

'Why? What for?'

'The sunset, of course. You shouldn't miss it.'

Hand in hand, we raced back to our meeting place while blue darkness arrived early. Flickering orange lights became visible within some of the shuttered apartments, the sun now casting a warm sand glow over the buildings. We reached Fountain Street just in time to watch the seawater snatch all remaining daylight, becoming a pale opal, before it appeared to fall asleep. Nan's smile shone like a star in the darkness and I was afraid to speak, reluctant to break this spell.

'Don't you want us to go anywhere, Harry?'

'Where?' An answer was obviously expected.

'Near here? Saturday?'

'Yes! The arch.'

It was here that we had shared our first kiss just two days earlier. We began to walk along St. Sebastian Street, skirting the edge of the sea, heading for the gunpost. A comfortable heat remained in the air and we ambled slowly, in no particular hurry, while day passed through the doorway into sudden night.

'This used to be different as well,' Nan rested her head against my shoulder. 'Used to be a lighthouse here, much better. That's how I like to think of it.'

We turned a corner, the three arches barely visible in thickening blackness. Under the furthest one, beneath the cool belly of stone, our tongues met tentatively, searching, learning. I could feel the backs of her front teeth, hot, wet ridges of palate. I didn't want to let her go. I didn't want to move from the spot.

'You,' she whispered. 'Where did you come from?'

I didn't know how to reply.

Nan had another plan for our evening, when we later visited a small café that she had discovered on Merchants Street.

'I've never eaten there, but it looks so nice every time I pass. I've never had anyone to take me,' she explained.

The dignified hush of this street made a welcome change to the suffocating rabble of Strait, and the Gut. We passed nobody; no crowds of drunken soldiers, no groups of painted women, and inside the café was empty.

'You didn't have to book us a private restaurant,' I joked, delighted to watch her smile. She looked so pure, so lovely, and too good for the likes of me. I had never met anyone to compare with Nan.

Our table was garnished with a sunflower in a sea-blue vase, bright paintings of the island adorning the walls. It was spotlessly clean, the proprietor a proud, bustling little woman, ably assisted by her young daughter. There were six tables packed tightly together, the kitchen hidden to the rear.

The smell of cooking was delicious.

I ordered the fish of the day, which transpired to be a generous chunk of tuna, and Nan ate homemade ravioli. While I enjoyed a bottle of beer, she chose to drink lemonade. I had never seen her touch a drop of alcohol. The conversation never wavered, and our hands met over the table.

'That was great Nan, the best meal I've had in ages.' My eyes caught on the thin gold chain about her neck, that I remembered so well from the weekend. 'What's your necklace?'

She released one of my hands, reaching for the chain, and I caught sight of the birthmark on her chest. My heart skipped a beat, surging with sudden desire. Nan withdrew a gold cross from somewhere close to her breasts.

'I'm a Catholic, Harry. I always wear it.'

The night was perfect, and it was with some reluctance that I escorted Nan back to her lodgings. I tried to walk as slowly as possible, choosing a route that I knew to be far from direct. I still had so much to say to her, the time had passed so swiftly. When I bent to kiss her goodnight, she placed one hand firmly onto my chest.

'Aren't you coming in?'

'Are you sure?' This time, my heart beat as swift as rapids. I had only ever slept with two women.

'Yes.' She took firm hold of my hand, pushed open the door, and led the way inside. 'I want you to stay tonight, but just wait here for a moment.'

The door was closed softly and she was gone, leaving me alone in a narrow, anonymous corridor. It was an uncomfortable, anxious wait, hoping that nobody else should appear. What could I say, to explain my presence? It was useless – I could think of no believable excuse. I was only capable of thinking about her and paced quietly, up and down, until I heard her voice.

'You can come in now.'

Nan had already taken off her clothes. I knew this because the first thing I saw was her dress folded neatly over the back of a chair. Beneath this, a glimpse of white underwear.

She sat upright in bed, which actually comprised of a mattress placed directly onto the floor. Arms hugging both knees, her bare shoulders were visible above a plain white sheet. The fine gold cross remained about her neck, disappearing down and under the cover. The room was small and bare, space only for a tiny wardrobe and drawers, yet I could not imagine anything more ideal.

'Hello, Harry,' I liked the way she spoke my name, as if sharing a secret.

Nan had positioned two small candles on the floor next to the bed, and a pale crescent moon shone weakly through the open window. The room smelled of her perfume. She lay back and watched as I removed my khaki uniform, feeling none of the nerves that I would have expected. Without hesitation, I climbed into bed and Nan's arms.

I held her close, our bodies stretched out in full contact, trying to touch everywhere. White heat crackled between us and I could feel her pressing against me, her stomach slender and taut. When we kissed, her tongue probed deep in my mouth. Determined to leave no part of Nan untouched, I began exploring her body with my lips.

I kissed the smoothness of her neck, the gold chain, taking the weight of the cross between my teeth. Stroking my fingers over the blood red birthmark, I ran my tongue along its continents and oceans, lapping the shorelines and mountains. Her own map of the world. She pushed her head back onto the pillow, sighing, and I continued down, taking my time.

Returning to Nan's face and more kissing, my own tongue now deep and frantic, I was aware of a scalding heat when finally entering her. We loved for a long time before collapsing, knotted together. I could not distinguish where one body ended and the other began, stroking what I believed to be Nan's leg.

'Harry,' she whispered, 'You told me you were a gentleman. So how come I'm lying on my back with you on top of me?' She kissed me on the lips.

'I can't really explain that. You've got me there.'

'You men, you're all the same.'

'We're not Nan, we're not.'

When I thought that she had fallen asleep, my finger traced indelible words onto her back. 'I love you.' She pressed backwards, against me, and I knew that I was finally in the right place in the world. It had certainly taken me long enough. I wrapped my arms about her, pulling her close, determined to never let go. I closed my eyes and attempted to dream of our future.

When it was time to leave, I propped myself up to kiss Nan on the forehead. I hadn't been able to sleep, simply content to lie in the dark and consider this newfound good fortune.

'Hello you. Nan?'

She twisted her body, getting both legs caught up in the sheet. Her breasts were uncovered, moist with perspiration, and I bent to kiss these in turn. Only then, she opened her eyes.

'Harry. Was I asleep?' Dark hair fell over her face, into her mouth.

'Yes. I didn't want to wake you. You looked so relaxed, but I'd better go now. It's nearly morning.'

I kissed her once more, and felt her hand reach to take hold of the back of my head. She would not let me leave so easily.

'I don't want you to, Harry. Stay.'

'Neither do I, but I've got to.'

She raised herself onto one elbow, to look at me properly.

'I feel good, thanks to you. Stay a little longer.'

'I really can't, I'm sorry. And there's something I've got to tell you.' I had been putting this moment off, in fear of jeopardising everything, but this was no longer possible. My throat felt so dry and I swallowed hard before continuing to speak. 'I'm getting transferred today, to the hospital in M'tarfa. I would have told you sooner but...'

Nan stopped me, a warm hand placed over my mouth.

'Harry, that's great news. I'm being sent there too!'

'Really? When?' I was filled with such tremendous happiness, and beginning to see omens everywhere. What's more, all of them were good. 'That's brilliant.'

'They haven't told me yet, but it's definitely going to happen. Soon.'

Leaving Nan's quarters, the day was already a hot one. There was not a cloud to be seen in the deep blue sky. I walked back to Sliema with the light, easy steps of a man in love.

CHAPTER TWO

It was a summer of fire in the sky, red wine, but most of all love. I knew right from the beginning that this was no ordinary affair - it was far greater than that. I loved Nan completely, with every tendon, muscle, and nerve in my body. With every drop of my blood. I had no choice. I loved with the absolute security that it could never end; this was no Straight Street relationship, and I understood right from the beginning that love does not have to stop. Not ever.

I was stationed on the small island of Malta, deep in the heart of the Mediterranean. Conditions did not seem so bad at the beginning, for civil rationing had not yet kicked in. No real shortages were evident. It was still possible to buy food, alcohol, and tobacco, in town; the local red wine surprisingly good. I quickly developed a taste for the Blue Label beer, not least to avoid the foul taste of our chlorinated water supply. After arriving, however, the thing that I enjoyed most about the island was its capital, Valletta.

It struck me immediately as a sweaty city - hot, dirty, and in no time at all I found myself delighted with the place. It was built on an impossibly grand scale, starting at the harbour, which had been my first real sight from the sea. This great hulk rose sheer out of the body of water, a solid mass of grey stone topped with elaborate spires, gunposts, and domes. In the distance, a cathedral flamed golden in the late afternoon sun. Flocks of white birds darted about the clear sky, the green sea no longer galloping about us. I had never seen anything like it, and Valletta excited me.

Beyond the harbour, I quickly discovered the city stretched outwards in a grid-iron plan of intersecting streets.

The principal artery, Kingsway, ran from an imposing gateway at one end of town, threading its imperious way down to Fort St. Elmo and the sea. All main squares and important buildings connected onto this. Kingsway never failed to remind me of a giant centipede, with roads falling from it like legs.

Parallel and next to Kingsway ran Strait, a dark, narrow street awash with numerous bars, clubs, and cafes. We called it the Gut, and nightlife for most of the servicemen was centred here. It was invariably crammed with jostling khaki and leathered faces, and transport was always laid on to and from the barracks.

Valletta was certainly fine, but the journey to the island had been an altogether different experience. After training was completed at Boyce Barracks in Hampshire, my company had been transferred to a base in Scotland. We were stationed in huts erected within the Earl of Dalkeith's estate outside Edinburgh, the main house now converted into a military hospital. The men were excited and ready for action, but not a single duty was allocated our way. It was a frustrating wait, the war tantalisingly close and yet still denied to us.

Stories began to spread like disease concerning where we were headed. Europe was the number one possibility, with Africa a close second. I soon learned that wherever a group of soldiers is gathered, there are at least as many rumours. On the third day we were issued with tropical kit, so at least we knew it would be somewhere hot. Another tortuous nine days were to pass in this manner.

We were finally mustered on the twelfth night, packed into lorries to Edinburgh, then loaded onto trains to Gourock on the Clyde. In this confusion of men, I found myself assigned to a French liner, the *Louis Pasteur*. It was a young lad with a spotty face who showed me to my cabin.

'Not a bad ship this one, sir. Been converted all right, better than some of them.' He spoke with a child's voice.

'Any idea where we're going?' It remained the first question on all of our lips.

'Don't know any more than you on that one, sir. Can tell you about the ship, though.' He continued chatting happily. 'She was one of the last to escape before Jerry occupied the Channel ports. Been refitted as a troop carrier, even got a hospital onboard. You're the nurse, right?'

'That's right.' I followed him quickly along wood-panelled corridors, down ornate stairways, descending steadily into the bowels of the ship. The air was getting warmer, and smelling of engine oil.

'Nurse in charge, I should say! There's just you. Got your own cabin, for that. I have to share mine with three others. Gets a bit stale in there, I can tell you. Here we are then.'

He stopped outside a dark door, reaching to grab hold of the shiny brass handle and opening it inwards.

'Your new home, sir. Hope you like it. I'll be around later, but got a few more to direct. Hospital's next door if you want to take a look. 'Bye then, sir.'

He disappeared in a clatter of enthusiastic footsteps, hurrying back to the deck. There would be many more men needing escort to allocated quarters.

I stepped into a cabin that was small but clean. It contained bunk beds and a single white cupboard for storage. I was pleased to have a porthole, a glimpse of the outside world, for I've always been claustrophobic. It would have to do. I flung my bag onto the lower bunk and went next door to investigate the hospital.

This was in fact a large cabin of white walls and gleaming silver metallic surfaces that resembled fish-bellies. We had space for eight casualties, to be nursed on bunk beds. I started opening the cupboards and drawers, to find out what materials I'd have available, to check where everything was stored.

The hospital was well stocked. I found boxes of hypodermic needles, a good range of medicines including antibiotics, and clear-labelled stores of blood. There were new scalpel blades, suture kits, sterile dressings. Stainless steel scissors remained in their packets; bottles of iodine and clove oil were arranged in precise formation. All that I required seemed to be there.

A sudden noise disturbed this investigation - the engines were starting below. Situated in the middle of the vessel, I would have to listen to the bronchitic cough, wheeze, and splutter, of the workings of the ship, but at least I had my own cabin. After several weeks of sleeping in a dormitory, this was indeed a great luxury.

The engines grew noisier, and I knew that we must be close to departure. At last, it was time to say goodbye to England. I made my way back to the deck for one last look at land, not knowing when or if I should return. Many of the men had the same idea, and there was definite excitement contained within the murmur of voices.

'So this is it then.'

A man on my right muttered to nobody in particular.

'This is it.' I mouthed a silent reply and found myself smiling. 'This is it,' I spoke aloud. The moment had taken so long to arrive and I was glad to be finally getting away. Ropes were cast off, the boat shuddered into action, and we were moving, sailing downstream into the blackness.

It seemed that I had only just fallen asleep when there was a loud knocking on my door. A man entered the room quickly, immediately flicking on the light switch.

'Sorry, sir, but you've got a patient. He's vomiting blood, I didn't want to wake you.'

He spoke fast, the words rushing out in a broad Scottish accent. The cabin light was a shock to my eyes, but I could not miss the stocky fellow with coarse red hair standing over my bed. I could tell that he was worried.

'Where is he?' I struggled out of the lower bunk, reaching for my trousers. It would be easier to sleep in my clothes, in future.

'I put him next door.'

'I'll be right with you, go check on him.'

He left the room. I fastened my shirt, snapping into alertness with each buttonhole. This was it, the start of my duties, and it felt so right. I was more than ready for this. Shoes were shoved on and I followed the Scot into the hospital next door.

The surgery was dazzling after the relative dark of my cabin, and it had already been christened into action. A young soldier sat in the middle of the floor, his shirt front soaked wet, vomiting blood into an overflowing steel kidney bowl. The floor was puddled in red. The man who had woken me stood next to him, one arm about his shoulders, supporting him. He looked relieved to see me.

'It's getting worse,' he stammered.

'When did it start?' I grabbed the kidney bowl, replacing it with a clean one, and poured the bloody mixture into the sink. It ran hot and sticky over my fingers, the smell so awful that I retched.

'Not sure. Maybe half an hour. We're sleeping next to

each other and he threw up all over the place.' The patient vomited again, groaning with the pain. 'Kept apologising, he did, but I told him not to worry.'

'How frequent is it?' I reached into the man's pocket for his record card.

'Every few minutes, it's not stopping. He's lost a lot of blood.'

Private William Smith was only nineteen. Blood group O, Rhesus positive. That was good news, the most common type. It was obvious he needed a transfusion as quickly as possible, to stabilise his condition.

'Right, can you help me get him onto a bed?' I turned to the patient. 'William, we're going to move you now.'

William nodded, listless. He had briefly stopped vomiting. The smell of the blood was cloying, sweet, and I was glad of the Scot's assistance. It gave me the confidence to get on with my work, to remain professional.

I rolled up William's sleeve, his left arm, before applying a tourniquet. It was useful that I had explored the surgery earlier. The veins were quick to show, liquid blue under the thin skin. An alcohol swab was wiped, my fingers careful to aim lateral to the tendon, and a needle selected. The Scotsman twisted away, his features suddenly pale.

I grabbed the arm, holding the skin tight, and pushed in with the steel. A flash of red, I was into a vein. Good. A container of blood was slowly emptied and we watched our patient improve. He stopped retching, the colour returned to his face. A drip was then secured, and I made sure he was rehydrated.

'Can I go now, Doc?' the Scot enquired. 'I've seen enough blood for the one night, right enough. He's looking better already.'

'Of course. And thanks for the help. Goodnight.'

With the patient in a stable condition, I swabbed the surgery methodically with disinfectant. The needle was wiped clean, for it would have to be re-used, and a spirit lamp flamed over its surface.

Returning to the deck, I discovered we had joined with a convoy. A faint wash of light dripped into the night sky, and I could make out seven other ships. The *Louis Pasteur* sailed in the second row, her movements graceful and steady. It was definitely a relief to breathe in the cool salt air.

We left the convoy after one day, to proceed alone. The ocean now kicking and bucking, many of the men began to suffer from seasickness. Many others were sick at the sight and smell of this, and I was glad to have nursing duties to keep me busy. I preferred to spend my time in the surgery.

The second patient had fallen and cut his forehead open, unused to the rolling motion of the ship. He was a tough Geordie and refused any anaesthetic, allowing me to stitch him up in thick, generous black thread. This could be removed later, after docking. We still had no idea where we were heading.

I prescribed antibiotics and clove oil for dental infections, medicine for stomach bugs, and enjoyed plenty of stitching practice as a procession of the men fell over. Private William Smith recovered quickly and was soon discharged from the hospital. He was sorry to leave me, getting used to having his own cabin.

My duties went well, but I noticed how life onboard seemed a particularly subdued experience for most of the men. This surprised me after the initial exuberance that I had witnessed on conscription. Walking along the dark-wooded passageways, there was little conversation amongst the soldiers, their heads nodding forwards in attempted rest. They were beginning to understand how we could actually be sunk and killed at any moment, for enemy submarines patrolled these waters. It was better to remain silent than spread such fears.

Nobody was able to change clothes, and an odour soon became evident, later characteristic of these men. It was the smell of leather and gun oil, of fatigue and rising fear. We were steaming relentlessly away from past lives and identities, away from our homes, but this only made me feel glad.

The *Louis Pasteur* changed direction, heading east into a warm wind. Soon, the long flat shadow of a coastline was spotted ahead, and we were informed that this was Africa. Men began to gather on deck simply to stare, for most of us had never left Britain. The dark stain on the horizon was an exotic sight, and we'd all heard the stories about how the native women wore no clothes. We hoped for a glimpse of this nakedness. Physical training sessions were arranged on the deck in an attempt to keep us fit, but sunbathing became the more popular activity.

We changed direction once more, this time sailing north while keeping the coast in view on our right. The sea became wild and strong, a tangle of currents and undertow, and the men continued to experience sickness. This situation did not improve, and even those who had been previously unaffected could be struck down at any moment. I remained happily immune, and again made sure that those most seriously affected did not become dehydrated. If I remained below decks, I missed the worst of this spectacle.

On the fourth day of the voyage, another land shadow was spotted ahead. We aimed directly for it, crowds of men collecting on the decks, until houses and roads could be distinguished. The *Louis Pasteur* glided as smoothly through the Straits as a new scalpel through soft flesh, and we dropped anchor in Gibraltar harbour. It was excellent to be moored against solid ground, but there were orders to obey and nobody was allowed onshore. We had to suffer another frustrating wait, staring enviously at all the people on land until darkness fell heavily into the sea.

I had not slept well on the ship, despite my regained privacy. There was still too much to think about, and the nursing duties kept me alert. I was forgetting about England, deliberately, and trying to prepare for the service ahead. It did not help that nobody had yet told us of our final destination.

In youth, I had been troubled with a recurring dream. This had started with the stress and uselessness of unemployment, disappeared for a long while, but now it chose to return.

In this dream, the first thing I am aware of is absolute silence and I know that the world must be dead. I am walking home on my own, past row upon row of identical grey houses, until eventually arriving at Park Street in Folkestone, where I was born. I climb two steps to the front door before discovering that I cannot find my keys.

I suddenly realise that I've been followed and someone is standing on the step right behind me. Cold hands reach out to stretch gently around my neck and I hear a voice mutter something indiscernible. It's my father, I think, and am unafraid, believing myself the victim of one of his drunken jokes. And then I hear his voice, but from inside the house.

'Is that you, Harry?'

The hands tighten rapidly and it's at this moment I invariably wake in a panic.

A horrible dream, it had always been a signpost to bad times ahead. I'd hoped to have left it behind, and worried what it might signify.

We remained in Gibraltar for two days, the men becoming increasingly restless. Still, nobody was allowed onshore which seemed particularly unfair on those soldiers who were seasick. Moored in the harbour made no difference to them, they continued to throw up and feed the shoals of tiny silver fish gathered about the boat. Our washing facilities were restricted, and the stench on the boat became dreadful. Of course, this sickness was in part related to fear.

I saw the Scotsman again, an entertaining chap by the name of Kerr. He told me he came from Glasgow, the best city in the world.

'Been busy, eh Doc?'

We stood together on the deck, Kerr careful to remain in the shade.

'On the way over I was. Nothing much now.'

'You'll be glad of that, eh? I'm missing ma home and ma pals. Could do wi' a good night, blow off some steam. Where do you stay, pal?'

'Sorry?'

'Where do you live?'

'London. But I'm originally from Folkestone. I moved there to study and ended up staying there.'

'A woman, eh?'

'You're right.' I joined him in the shade. Clouds shaped like animals raced over our heads, the heat stifling. I watched a white rabbit overtake a flock of plump sheep.

'So where do you think we're headed, pal? I hope it's not Africa - wasn't made for the heat, me.'

'Wish I knew. I just want to get there now. What's it like in Glasgow then? Why's it so good? I've never been, only to Edinburgh.'

He looked aghast.

'You're missing out, pal. It's a grand old city, much better than that snooty look down their noses at you Edinburgh. Got a lucky charm from ma local there - it's a piece of the bar, to keep me going 'til I get back.'

Kerr rummaged in his shirt pocket to locate a perfectly cut square of dark wood. He gave it an extravagant kiss before replacing it with care. He patted his shirt to make sure that it had not been dropped, that it was safe.

'Sweet, eh? Barman's going to stick it back after all this is over. Everybody's got one, eh? A lucky charm. So what do you carry?'

It was my turn to place a hand into my thick canvas shirt pocket. From this, I produced a small plaster of Paris teddy bear replete with blue bow tie. Kerr grinned.

'A woman, eh?'

'My first girlfriend, Dot Golding. You're right though, pretty much every patient I've seen has been holding onto something.'

'Aye, some of the men been complaining there's not enough action, but it's been enough for me all right. I'm in no hurry to get shot.'

'Me neither.'

That night, two hundred of us were ordered to transfer to an Australian destroyer, *Nestor*. Others were billeted on *Fearless* and *Manchester*. We had been on Gibraltar too long, it was a rushed job, but I felt relief to move on and leave my quarters onboard the *Louis Pasteur*. She was considered too big a target to sail into the Mediterranean. *Nestor* was a lot smaller in comparison, and I now had to share a cabin with another nurse. Lance Hadley was a big man, great tufts of black hair growing from out of his nostrils and ears, a heavy smell of sweat to the man. We shook hands and he was able to tell me our final destination. Malta.

'Try and get some rest, Harry. We're not leaving 'til morning. Jesus, I'm getting too old for this game.'

Lance was asleep within minutes, keeping me awake with his foghorn snores. The cabin was a miniature version of the one I'd left behind, only without a porthole. I lay on the top bunk, thinking of nothing but the island of Malta. Where was it? Why were we going there? What was it like? Basically, I knew nothing.

A red sun shimmied high into the sky when *Nestor* cast off in the morning. We sailed alone, heading back into the Atlantic. White caps jabbed at our stern, but the Australian crew seemed far happier on the rough water. Lance showed me around the hospital and when I returned to the deck we had joined with a new convoy. A dozen grey vessels rose and fell together, like the keys of a piano playing the music of the sea. All day, we waited; I was getting used to this. Large white gulls hovered above the decks, hungry for any scraps of food, and Lance was shat upon right on the head. I told him my mum would have said that was lucky, but he didn't share this opinion.

After the curtain of night closed tight, we returned to the Mediterranean. It was still possible to see lights shimmering like summer flowers on both sides, in Spain and North Africa, a welcome sight after the blackout in London. I imagined that I could hear foreign voices drifting out on the wind, that I could smell exquisite tropical dishes. Life was suddenly filled with new possibilities.

A vibration in the air disturbed these thoughts. Heads appeared on the deck, inquisitive, as this turned into a drone. When it became a scream, and the alarm sound detonated, a frantic activity infected the vessel. We were under our first attack.

I was running towards my station at the rear of the ship when an almighty bang exploded from the almost silent sea. A black shadow hurtled inches over my head - a depth charge. More would follow. The air itself felt swollen to bursting as the noise of attack quickly intensified. Somebody shouted 'submarine', blinding flashes lit up the night sky. One of our convoy was struck, *Fearless*. I knew some of the men onboard.

Nestor moved alongside, to provide cover, and I watched the convoy regroup to protect her. It was hard to locate the source of this attack, a confusion of noise and sharp daggers of light. Our guns were firing at something with deafening bursts of accuracy, and *Fearless* had managed to remain afloat. Shadows of her men were illuminated on the decks, waiting for our help.

Finally, thankfully, the chaos of battle subsided. The crew of *Fearless* was swiftly moved onto different vessels, although not *Nestor*, and she was left on her own, listing dangerously.

'This'll be some sight Harry.' Lance stood next to me.

'Why?'

'Got to sink her now.' Explosions sounded from one of our convoy. 'Stop her falling into enemy hands.'

A heavy crumpling sound was heard when *Fearless* burst into flame. Night became day and, slowly, her bow turned up. She disappeared gently, elegantly, into the ink-black water.

Lance and I returned to the surgery where, to our surprise,

we discovered that there were no casualties yet onboard.

After days without action, the men were excited. The Australians had seen all this before, but those from the *Louis Pasteur* were high on adventure. The talk raged about *Fearless* going down, how we had saved her crew. We knew things would be hotting up now. Sleep proved elusive and unnecessary.

It was early morning when we were relocated by enemy reconnaissance planes. Everything happened at once, with submarines joined by dive and torpedo bombers in attacking the convoy. In the muddle of sudden battle, *Manchester* was now hit and rolled badly. We watched in dismay as she was forced to leave us, turning and limping backwards in the direction of Gibraltar. Enemy pilots broke away, trying to finish her off. Her chances did not look good. She was obviously in no shape to reach Malta and I hoped she would make it on her own. My pal Kerr was onboard.

We now had our first casualties to treat, mainly caused by the shower of shrapnel. Cuts were stitched up, bleedings staunched, and one man needed bandages over both his eyes. Something had struck him to cause a nasty mess, which Lance and I could do little about. He would need further treatment on the island.

Now, I watched with interest how the eyes of the patients shrank back into their heads, withdrawing from the war. This spoke to me of loss, a craving for homes and loved ones who may never be seen again, an anticipation of killing. It was all suddenly very real. The sea around us appeared to shiver, mirroring these fears, as men acquired the eyes of mortality.

Nestor somehow continued on her way, and on the third night Italian biplanes joined the assault. Lance had told me how the Italian pilots were not known for their bravery, but these planes flew in terribly close, risking the bursts of anti-aircraft fire. It was almost impossible to pry eyes away and run for cover, with more and more men drawn to watching the awful spectacle. The injuries we treated grew worse, shrapnel sometimes embedded so deeply into bodies that it was impossible to remove. With so many bombs, bullets, and shells flying, the roar of battle was terrifying. Perforated eardrums became another source of admission, and I almost envied the men their subsequent period of deafness.

Italian E-boats became prevalent, and these small unmanned torpedo craft attempted to penetrate our protective screen. *Nestor* sailed on the outside of the convoy, covering the merchantman boats that carried supplies, firing relentlessly. It was during this night that two of these evil, black craft managed to break through.

Two ships in our convoy received direct shuddering hits, before exploding into a strangely beautiful blossom of fireworks. Bright flames shot hundreds of feet high, and there must have been survivors in the water because I heard their cries. They did not last long, the flames soon reached them. No semblance of boats remained.

This night, I saw my first bodies floating face down in the sea, the loneliest sight in the world. The Mediterranean of my boyhood dreams had become a sea of darkness and nightmares, a sea of death where only ghosts could be found swimming. I stood on the deck and a man groaned loudly, stumbling against me, knocking us both from our feet. I caught him as we went down, a little fellow, searching immediately for the cause of his injury. My lap felt suddenly warm and I located the problem right then. A skull wound.

'Got to turn you over pal.' I hoped he could hear me.

As I adjusted my weight to move him, the soldier juddered twice. A low moan escaped his lips before the body went unmistakably limp. I looked at his face to make sure, felt for the carotid pulse in the neck. Nothing. He was dead, a mere boy. With horror, I recognised the face of my first patient; it was Private William Smith.

Blinding white angel light reflected in his eyes as another of our convoy was hit. This time it was close, the ship next to *Nestor*. I had stopped hearing sounds, aware only of what I could see. Two shadows jumped into the water above the source of the blast, preferring to take their chances that way. Poor bastards.

The ship did not go down. No fire shot into the sky, and I realised that *Nestor* was pulling closer. We were going to help. It was the *Sydney Star*, another of the merchantmen. Her cargo must be important. I lowered William gently to the floor.

Nestor drew alongside, but some of the *Star's* lifeboats had got stuck, obstructing the way. It was one of our Australian crew who immediately climbed over the side, hacking away at the holding gear, while the battle petered out. The lifeboats dropped into the sea and *Nestor* was level with *Star*. Glancing away, I saw that the remainder of the convoy continued without us.

A gangplank was positioned and *Star's* crew rushed onto *Nestor*, faces glistening pale with moonlight. I didn't know where we could fit them, but obviously they couldn't be left behind. The *Star* remained afloat; her condition did not appear to have worsened. I carried William Smith to the mortuary, and Lance told me later how the Captain had placed a prize crew onboard, in an attempt to save the cargo. The torpedo had hit a hold containing flour; she'd been lucky not to go up like the other two.

It was inevitable that we soon found ourselves under further attack. An enemy plane spotted us and arrowed away. We thought we were in the clear until the reinforcements arrived, an angry buzzing in the dark sky. Suddenly, groups of high and low-level bombers were swarming about us, like buzzards in for the kill. *Nestor* cast off the tow rope and began to circle the merchantman, surrounding her with a blanket of silver fire. We were going to go down fighting, and I watched two of the planes drop smoking into the sea.

Light began to drizzle into the day, the edge of the sky touched with pure blue light. Canon shells and bullets tore through our side plates, while Lance and I had more casualties to treat. More wounds to clean up, more stitching, more dressings. More fatalities. We were fast becoming soldiers as we grew increasingly aware of what we were able to face. We would prove good soldiers once we had learned to accept death with indifference. And so we carried on with our work, increasingly covered with blood, as *Nestor* struggled forwards. It took some time to realise that the noise of attack had abated and, when the patients were stable, I took my chance to return to the deck.

The sun shone bright in a sky banded with thin wisps of white cloud. The Captain was checking our damage; he was a man and a half, a real leader, according to Lance. I couldn't understand how we remained afloat, watching the crew sweep overboard a jangle of nuts, bolts, and rivets, which had been shaken loose from our plates, but he appeared to be unconcerned. He saw me and he waved.

'So, how's it going down below? All under control?'

'Yes, sir. Now it is.'

'Good. Those bastards set my bed on fire with their damn

incendiary bullets. Didn't get us though. We'll make it yet.'

I nodded as he continued his inspection. We'd made it this far without the convoy, but there was still a way to go. The sea was calm beneath us, enjoying a doze. Wished I could do the same, but my head was buzzing with noise. My clothes rigid with dried blood, I managed to take a quick wash.

The attacks continued, blending into one long mess of battle. The wounded merchantman had now become the main target, and *Nestor* endured countless near misses on her behalf. Seawater cascaded in a wild dance over our deck, repeatedly blown into the air from the blast of falling bombs. It continued to be busy in the surgery, and I detected a further change creeping into the eyes of our patients; they would secretly study each other, searching for faces of the imminent dead. They tried to understand the situation, how much circumstances had changed. We were all living from moment to moment now.

An excited shout reached the surgery when *Edinburgh* had been spotted, coming to assist us. By the time Lance and I climbed into the daylight, six RAF planes also provided air cover. It could only mean one thing - we had nearly made it. The Italians were not so brave when the fight was more evenly matched.

It was the time before dusk, the light a little uncertain, when Malta finally appeared. A cheer was born on our decks and I felt the greatest pleasure to be approaching dry land. Finally, we would be allowed off the ship for the first time in ten days. The fortified battlements and watchtowers of the harbour looked magnificent, and I felt for Dot's bear with gratitude. So far, my luck had held out.

Entering the still waters of the harbour, I spotted the remainder of our convoy already at anchor. People waved from the stone walls and we were happy to wave back, especially those men on the towed *Star*. Sporadic bouts of cheering heralded our arrival on the island. So this was Malta, July 25, 1941. I was a long way from home. It was exactly what I'd wanted.

CHAPTER THREE

My trials for the night were only just beginning. I lost a toss with Lance, and had to take charge of the baggage party. He was particularly delighted because this was a tough job on any occasion, having to transfer all the gear off *Nestor* and then into army lorries. Four days and nights of little or no sleep, attack after bloody attack, we all just wanted to rest. It seemed a harsh call as we passed each other numerous heavy boxes, and the red-faced young officer attempting to hurry us up was easily ignored.

It took hours. I watched my colleagues climb wearily into the open back of a small truck to be driven away, and was left to follow in one of the loaded vehicles. My only company was the short, fat, Maltese driver who appeared to have more hair coming out of his ears than on top of his head. He apparently spoke no English, each of my questions met with an indifferent shrug of the shoulders. I didn't like him, his scruffy vest, or his dirty shorts.

The shirt stuck onto my back when sitting inside the cab, and I felt in desperate need of a clean. The engine fired into deafening, bone-shaking life on the second attempt, and we were off, bouncing and juddering along the sea front. It was completely black outside, except for our headlights. I was dog-tired and thinking only of sleep when a familiar siren kicked off, heralding the start of yet another attack. This time it was targeted on the harbour. The air exploded with fire and noise, my driver slammed on the brakes, flung open his door, and ran away. I never saw him again.

I had no idea where I was, or where we were going. A heavy rain of shrapnel began to pop in the air, striking the ground about the truck. There was only one thing I could do without abandoning the charge - I opened my door and crawled quickly beneath the vehicle.

Sprawled on a dusty, bumpy road, my vantage point provided a surprisingly clear view of the action. With the harbour illuminated by a tangle of searchlights, each beam cutting slits in the stomach of night, I watched the sky transform into a mad scribble of dark red, green, and light red lines. The constant flashes and explosions became mesmerising, but I remember glancing at my watch. Quarter to five in the morning.

I lay without moving, thinking about the blood rushing throughout my own body, red wine coursing along dark alleys, the quiet places, and I could feel nothing. Numbed with exhaustion, I simply admired the insane beauty of it all. It was almost a disappointment to hear the all clear ring out, another unsuccessful attack. For a few long minutes, I remained still. It was an effort to squirm out, to resist sleep a little longer.

The lorry had sustained one gashed tyre, and I had no choice but to stay put. Sounds of activity drifted up from the docks, but the sky remained dark. Considering Lance tucked up, snoring, in bed, brought on evil thoughts. I knew I should have called heads, and didn't feel so lucky now. It seemed ages before two army gunners approached, riding a motorbike and sidecar.

'What's up here mate?' The man on the bike removed his helmet revealing a handsome, boyish face. I explained quickly what had happened.

'Bad luck, eh? Italians tried to take the harbour, but intelligence must have known about it. Soon sent them running. Anyway, we'll have to leave you here, but I'll get help sent along.'

Some half an hour later, I was delivered exhausted to a hospital outside of Sliema. A nurse wearing a blue dress handed me a pint mug of tea that looked too good to be true. I was hot, dry, my uniform filthy with dust, and I gulped greedily before the taste suddenly registered. It was foul, disgusting, an unforgettable first taste of the chlorinated water on the island.

'You do get used to it,' she touched my arm.

'Really? I couldn't possibly have a beer could I? It's been a long night.'

A bottle of Blue Label was found from somewhere, and this was much better. From that moment, I decided to drink it whenever possible. Briefing was arranged for later that morning and I was shown to an empty bed. Sleep did not come easy. In the steamed heat of the room, I could feel cascades of sweat evaporating from my body like insects crawling all over my skin.

I woke early, restless. My dreams had again been disturbed, of Park Street, guns, and bombs. Of Private William Smith. It felt good to leave them behind.

The room was bright, an orange sun shining directly through the closed window. No wonder I was so hot. It took a few moments to register where I was, but I knew straight away it wasn't the boat; that was something to be grateful for. I tried to recount events of the previous night, to remember my instructions for today. Had to report to the Major, that was it, 10.00 hours. I looked at my watch. 09.30, good, but I couldn't afford to be late. I had slept in my clothes, which remained covered in an icing of dust.

It was a struggle to climb out of bed, my limbs stiff with complaint from the baggage party. I groaned to bend for my shoes, then hobbled painfully towards the door.

'Where's the bathroom, mate?'

A soldier hurried past. He turned to answer.

'Straight down the corridor, first left.' He rushed on.

I walked slowly, unsure of solid ground after the rolling movement of the ship. My head continued to sway, hesitant to adapt, and I needed to steady myself with one hand against the wall. My footsteps echoed weakly on the smooth wooden floor, as if part of me was missing.

Inside the washroom, a line of four white sinks dazzled the eyes, topped with four small mirrors. Thick swathes of yellow light streamed through two open windows, bouncing shards of brightness across the room. The floor was slippery with other people's wash-water, but I didn't care. I strode to the nearest basin, turned on the tap, and noticed my face in the mirror.

Eyes ringed with dark shadows, pale, a forehead ploughed with wrinkles; I looked old. It was my father's frown that stared back at me. The water was freezing cold when I plunged my head beneath the surface, scalp shrinking in complaint, but I remained in this position for as long as I could bear.

Quickly, I lifted my head, rubbing my hair with a towel that someone had discarded. It smelled damp, foreign, and unpleasant. I gazed in the mirror once more, and still a stranger looked back.

After wandering along several identical corridors, asking numerous directions, I reported to the Major at 09.55. Five minutes early. His Maltese secretary sat outside the office, dark and plump, her eyes resembling little black coals. Caught up in a possession of typing, her desk blocked the narrow passageway.

'I'm here to see the Major.'

'Your name?' she didn't look up, barely broke her rhythm on the shiny metallic keys.

'Fisher, Harold. I arrived last night.'

With reluctance, she tutted to a stop and ran a short, stubby finger down a sheet of white paper. Upside down, I spotted it rest on my name.

'Yes. Major Merryweather's expecting you. You'll have to wait here.'

She recommenced her typing, able to ignore me once again. I stood in the corridor while time dripped past with agonising sloth. My mind, which had been a snarl of loose thoughts, began to tighten into memories of home. London. Continued relief to get away.

'Get in here, now!'

A voice like gunshot burst into the corridor. I ran to open the door, salute at the ready, feeling trepidation at this anger. The Major was standing behind his desk, eyes narrowed, shouting at a startled little dog that scurried to his side. He looked surprised to see me, perhaps embarrassed.

'Who are you? What do you want?' The words came quickly. He spoke in a well-educated voice.

'Fisher, sir. Reporting for duty.'

'Yes, yes. But why did you come rushing in like that?'

'I thought you called me, sir.'

'Why?'

'You said, "Get in here, now".'

The Major, who had been looking particularly stern-faced, allowed himself a chuckle.

'I see Fisher,' he continued, voice softened. 'Only I was shouting at this damn dog. His basket is under the desk, and I have to look after him today.'

'Sorry, sir. Shall I go back out?'

'No, no. Of course not. Sit down, man.'

The office was small and tidy, all papers lined in a meticulous straight line on the desk. It had a large window for the size of the room, and I could make out a deep band of blue behind the Major's head. On Malta, the sea would never be far away.

The Major himself was a short man, apparently in his forties, and wore silver-rimmed round spectacles. He had a trim brown moustache, dark hair greying markedly over both temples, his eyes intelligent and alert. He gestured to a chair positioned against the wall.

'I'm sure you must be tired.'

He perched behind the desk, movements agile, those of a younger man. Only then did I sit.

'Right, where to begin?' His eyes closed briefly, he swallowed noisily. 'I'm glad you've managed to join us. We heard you had a rough time of it?' Eyes on me, this was a question.

'Yes, sir. We did. I'm very glad to be here.' This was very true. It was a delight to be on solid ground once more.

'Well, tell me what you know about the island?'

'Not much, sir.'

I'd better put you in the picture, so you know what you're in for.' He spoke kindly, without any trace of condescension. 'We came under attack last year, with Italy and Britain at war. You know all that. Thought they could take the island in days, but they underestimated us. Dropped a lot of bombs, mind. You see, we need Malta to land planes flying between England and Egypt. They're planning a North African campaign now, so things are hotting up.

You'll be with us here at Sliema for a few days, but then we'll be sending you to the permanent holding company on the island. You'll be based at the 90th General Hospital, M'tarfa.'

'Where's that, Major?'

'Right in the middle of the island. But first we need you here, to help prepare the hospital ahead of receiving patients. Going to be busy soon - you've drawn a good one, Fisher. I suggest you familiarise yourself with the place today, and get yourself down to the Gut in Valletta. You've earned a night out, I should think.'

'Thank you, sir.'

'Right then' he stood up, 'my secretary will tell you where to report tomorrow.'

We shook hands and I turned to leave the office.

'Good luck, Fisher.'

His parting words did not inspire confidence.

Sliema stood on a hill overlooking the capital, Valletta. Outside the hospital, I watched a steady stream of people flowing down to enter the city. Yellow houses stretched between two impressive waterfronts from where I stood, one facing a wide inlet harbour, the second the Mediterranean.

I walked to Balluta Bay and the open water. Here shone the sea of my childhood dreams, heaving itself gently in and out of the many rock pools. The water flickered blue-green, like the wings of a dragonfly. I wanted to swim, but after the Italian attack of last night thought this might be rather foolish. Instead, I ambled slowly along hot, dusty streets, thinking about the truth of an old saying back home; only mad dogs and Englishmen would choose to be out in this heat.

Passing the occasional shop, a collection of churches, I eventually arrived at the harbour. Marsamxett it was called, not where we'd arrived. The wind whisked up a generous froth of water, clots of white surf breaking onto the rocks below me. In the distance, Valletta rose majestic from out of the blue. I could distinguish the cathedral spotted from *Nestor* more clearly, the full extent of the battlements. The Major was right; I should visit there tonight. In the afternoon, I managed to catch up on some much needed sleep.

An open lorry drove me and four others into Valletta, depositing us at the top end of Kingsway. My companions were all excited at the prospect of another night on Strait Street, the Gut, but I fancied exploring first. I wanted to get my bearings.

I walked past the Opera House on Kingsway, a majestic elaboration of white columns, statues, and frescoes. Regent Cinema was on the left, soldiers and their girls just coming out from an afternoon show. A lovely old library was positioned on the right. Kingsway certainly appeared impressive, a real change from England, and the heat was now more bearable. A cool breeze jostled and hurried along the street, fresh from the sea. It felt good. I'd just entered a large square when a voice called out my name.

'Harry Fisher! Blimey, what you doing out here?'

A hand waved from across the road and I recognised Dicky Fuller, an old pal from Folkestone.

'Dicky! Good to see you.'

We shook hands in the middle of the street. Dicky slapped me hard on the back.

'Harry Fisher, eh? Come on, I'll buy you a drink.'

Dicky had always been a slight fellow, maybe 5 ft. 8 ins. to my six feet, but he had definitely broadened out. His head no longer appeared too big for the body. His fine brown hair was cut short, green eyes twinkling from under heavy eyebrows. The thing about Dicky was his good humour; he'd always been popular back home. He'd also been a top dancer, winning many local prizes with his wife.

'You're looking well, mate.'

'I keep good health, Harry. Best present your parents can give you, eh?'

I thought about his Irish mother, a good, simple woman, in his own words. His father had been high up in the British Army, a born raconteur. As boys, he'd kept us fascinated with stories of service abroad in India, how he'd been a witch doctor in Africa. Dicky had inherited this gift of storytelling.

'I'll take you to the Services Club. You've been there before, right?'

'Only just got here. It's my first time out.'

He pinched my arm. 'Well, you're in for a treat then.'

We entered through a yellow stone doorway leading into the "Union Jack." It was a large bar. Thick clouds of smoke made it hard to see clearly and I struggled not to cough. The Victory V cigarettes on the island created one horrible stench.

'So, what will you have Harry? Beer?'

I nodded, scanning eyes about the room. It was crowded with soldiers, the atmosphere unmistakably of release, freedom, and excitement. A brown glass bottle was thrust into my hand. Blue Label.

'Well, cheers then!' We chinked our bottles together and I swallowed deeply. The cold liquid felt wonderfully soothing on the throat against the bitter smoke in the bar.

'So tell me how you got here then,' Dicky shouted.

'It wasn't easy.' I told him about *Fearless* and *Manchester*, the *Sydney Star*.

'Yeah, we'd heard you had a bad time of it. *Manchester*

made it back to Gibraltar anyway. I better get you another beer! Only just got here myself. I'm with the Buffs now, nearly got wiped out in France. They had to completely reform us. Anyway, cheers my friend!' We chinked bottles again. 'To Folkestone, eh?'

'To Folkestone. It's busy in here, Dicky. Is this normal?'

He smiled.

'Harold, you ain't seen nothing yet.' Dicky slapped me on the back again and roared with laughter. 'Come on, I'll show you somewhere else.' He emptied his bottle in a single gulp, and moved for the door.

'It's the girls, Harry,' he turned briefly. 'You want to see the girls.'

I was just in time to spot Dicky's head turn right and vanish through another doorway, entering into "The British Queen". When I managed to catch up he already held our beers.

'This one's for the girls, Harry! Drink up, and look around you.'

He was right. In every corner of the bar, groups of women stood chatting with soldiers. Their clothes revealed oceans of dark flesh, and many wore gaudy red lipstick. Eyes were dark, sultry, mysterious.

'Don't get women like that in Folkestone, eh? They're like buses out here, Harry. Never chase one, there'll always be another along in a minute!' He cackled noisily, whooping with glee; war obviously suited Dicky Fuller.

'Okay Harry, so what do you need to know? I'll show you the ropes.' His face frowned in concentration. 'Stinking heat's the first thing. Watch out for that. Be careful not to burn, although you'll soon get used to it. Haircuts every week out here, and nails grow something rotten. Get yourself some scissors. Flies'll drive you mad, too – have to learn to ignore them.'

I'd already noticed these on the island. Damn things wouldn't leave a person alone, diving in as relentlessly as our attackers.

'Got to watch out for all the churches - lording it over us! Ignore them, too. Many of the women are Catholic, but mostly it's only in name. Taxi carriage drivers…' He was in his stride now, the words racing furiously out. 'Shower of bastards the world over! Always agree on a price first, or they'll rob you blind. What's up Harry, you're as silent as a fish?'

'Nothing, Dicky. Just listening.' And watching all the women, which I did not care to admit. I was surprised to find them so attractive, and hadn't really expected to discover anything like the Gut.

'Good, good. So come on, ask me another one!'

'Tell me about the girls, Dicky.'

'Ah, yes, the girls. I was getting to them.' He cackled again. 'Just one thing to remember mate, many of them are Sherry Bandits and that's prostitutes to you and me. Always keep a hand on your money, and you've got to be careful not to catch something nasty. I tell you, they're Catholics only in name.'

I remembered the Captain of *Nestor* telling me how all but six of his crew had needed treatment for venereal diseases. There had been definite pride in his voice.

'But you'll be okay,' Dicky continued, smiling. 'You nurses, you can always get hold of the right medicines!'

Dicky's laugh was infectious and I chuckled with him.

'See anyone you like, Harry?'

'They're all good.'

'That's right. That's right.' He rested a hand on my

shoulder as we both studied the room. Some of the women could be seen perched on laps of the men, not one of them was left unattended.

'What about your wife, Dicky? Back home?' I regretted the words as soon as they were uttered, but he didn't seem in any way bothered.

'Another thing to remember, Harry. Minds are like parachutes mate, they only work when open. Things are different out here. It's all new.' He patted my shoulder. 'Don't forget that. So are you ready for another beer?'

We walked further up Strait, passing crowds of soldiers, exaggerated laughter, and raucous shouting. A woman wearing a short skirt smiled from a narrow doorway, blowing me a kiss. Cigarette smoke hung low in the alley and archways. The "Morning Star Club" appeared on our right.

'You'll like this Harry. It's one of the best.'

We pushed a way through to the bar.

'Two bottles Blue Label, mate,' Dicky shouted to the short Maltese barman. This beer tasted good. A woman immediately sidled up to us, her smile thick and sweet as honey. A vivid swipe of lipstick stuck to her upper teeth.

'Hello.' She spoke to both of us, hedging her bets. 'Having a good night? You look like real men to me.'

'Not wrong there, darling,' Dicky replied, immediately resting one hand against the curve of her bottom. She looked down and continued to smile, approving.

'Playing with fire tonight, are we?'

'So are you going to warm me up then?'

'Maybe.'

Dicky grinned, then pecked her on the cheek, the way you'd kiss an old lady.

'Can't tonight, love, sorry. Showing my pal the ropes, he's

new here. Come on Harry, let's get us a karozzin.'

He moved towards the door and I was happy to follow. The woman scowled as we rushed away and I shrugged, apologetic.

'Got to watch out for those ones, Harry.' Dicky waited for me outside. 'More edge than a broken piss pot! And I'm a gentleman anyway, not many of us left.' He laughed again. 'Come on, this way.'

He now disappeared up one of the tiny streets that I supposed would lead back onto Kingsway. One thing about Dicky that hadn't changed, he was always in a hurry. After my first beers in a long while, it was an unsteady rush to keep up with him, and there was little time to admire the ornate balconies hanging prettily over our heads. The air felt clean and fresh again after the nicotine choke of the Gut. It was suddenly quiet and dark, the revellers left behind and all local people wisely disappeared until morning.

Rounding the corner, Dicky was struggling awkwardly into a horse-drawn carriage. He appeared comical, all bony elbows and knees. Several other carriages waited patiently in line for hire, and these were the karozzins. Each had four large wheels lending an appearance of size, which quickly proved deceptive.

I clambered into the carriage while Dicky agreed on a fare, shouting instructions to the driver. We sat on facing horsehair-upholstered seats, our knees knocking repeatedly against each other.

'The grand tour tonight mate, first stop the Opera House.'

The carriage jerked into motion, trundling slowly away from the sea.

'You've got to get a woman in one of these, Harry. It's great. You can even shut yourselves in see?' He drew the canvas curtains that hung on either side. 'Women love a bit of romance, eh? Doesn't do you any harm. Look, there's the old Regent.' He pointed out of the window. 'I like to see a good film. Always cool inside, worth remembering.'

Kingsway was deserted after the bustle of Strait, all lights blacked out as they had been in London.

'Haven't met a woman who didn't love a ride in one of these, Harry. Worth every penny. Remember that, too! Look, there's the old Opera House. Lovely, isn't she?'

The building glowed luminous, pale with silver moonlight.

'It's beautiful, Dicky.'

'Not half, Harry. Like the women eh? Don't get 'em like this back in Folkestone.'

Dicky smiled with contentment, a flash of white in the dark carriage. The driver changed direction, heading downhill towards the harbour. We passed streets that appeared to be completely blocked with fallen stone, heaps of rubble piled dangerously high. It was hard to see in the poor light, the devastation appeared to be dreadful, but Dicky seemed unperturbed. He continued to talk with enthusiasm.

'There's a group of us going out on Saturday, Harry. See if you can come. One of them's a local girl, a nurse like you. Think you'll like her. Not like most of the others, a touch of class about her. Do you want to come along?'

'Not sure if I can yet, Dicky. I don't know my shifts, and I'm not really looking for someone.'

My personal life in England had enough problems without adding further complication immediately.

'Course not, Harry, but that's not really the point. Come anyway, it'll be fun. They're a good old bunch.'

Dicky suddenly rapped on the side of the carriage, shouting at the driver to stop. 'Do you fancy seeing a show now? There's everything out here, even women with dogs and bottle tricks.'

'Not really, thanks.' It was not for me.

'Suit yourself, mate. But I'll see you on Saturday. Union Jack again, about six if you can make it. Good seeing you, Harry. Cheerio.'

He rested one hand on my leg to launch himself from the carriage. I could hear his chuckle shrinking back along the dark, narrow streets as the driver turned around in his seat.

'Where now, then?'

'Sliema, please.' It was easier to go home. 'Balluta Bay.' Dicky's whirlwind of advice had left me exhausted, my mind wound tight as fishing twine. I was going to have that swim now, to help me to relax. When we reached streets that I recognised, I chose to walk the rest of the way.

The sea appeared to glow under moonlight, a phosphorescent opal. I hadn't noticed this on *Nestor*, but there had been too much going on. The bay was deserted and I stripped off all my clothes, arranging them into a tidy pile on the rocks. I waded quickly into the water's cool embrace.

Thanks to Dicky, I now had a working knowledge of Valletta and could see why the men enjoyed it. But I knew from the voyage and the Major that this wasn't an easy option. They'd seen plenty of action on the island, plenty more to come. I pulled deep strokes through the water before turning, floating, on my back.

Saturday night. The nurse. Of course I'd go if possible, but there was something about it that troubled me and I couldn't understand why. I listened to stones on the seabed click and slide over each other. Gazing up at the distant blackness, new stars now shone in the sky.

CHAPTER FOUR

In the morning, I found myself working with a bunch of Yorkshire men. Most of them came from Leeds, and as the Major had explained our duty was to ready the hospital in order to receive a greater number of patients. They were obviously expecting heavy casualties, a fact we didn't dwell upon.

The first job was a bad one, checking the bed frames for tiny bugs that seemed manifest on the island. A paraffin lamp was used to blast them clean. We joked that when supplies ran out, they'd get us doing this using sticks.

Next, in teams of two, the beds had to be positioned carefully so that none stood directly beneath windows or, more importantly, glass. It wasn't as simple as that, because the four legs each had to be placed into tins containing carbolic acid. There was a definite knack to this.

I was paired with Jeff Ellis, a sallow faced man with pale, sandy hair, and a dry wit. Jeff balanced the bed on two legs, holding the weight against him, while I positioned the tins. It was important not to overfill them, or they immediately spilled over. Once two legs had been sorted, the procedure was repeated by tilting the bed in the opposite direction. There was a lot of cursing to be heard as the tins refused to behave, spilling or shedding their contents repeatedly.

It didn't end there. Due to the hot weather, these containers required constant topping up. The smell was absolutely dreadful, a burning assault to both nostrils and throat. It hurt to inhale, seeming as if the memory of it would never disappear, we'd never be able to smell another thing. After this, the bed frames were liberally coated with grease, again to stop the bugs.

A second mattress was positioned underneath each bed. This was for when future air raids took place, to protect any patients who were unable to move. All remaining surfaces were swabbed meticulously with disinfectant.

Once one ward was completed, another followed. It was tedious work in the extreme, frustrating and mundane. Surely we'd been trained to do more than this, and I looked forward to my impending transfer. Paired with Jeff, we took notes of available stock on each ward, listing materials that were in short supply.

When Saturday arrived, I was off-duty and desperate for a night out. Dicky was just the man I needed to break the monotony of work, and a group of us from Sliema hopped into the back of a truck for the short drive to Valletta.

Walking into the Union Jack, I was twenty minutes early. The bar was already crowded, the air again thick with smoke, and I coughed immediately. I couldn't get used to those fags. I stood just inside the doorway, hoping for some fresh air while searching for my friend.

'Harry, we're over here!'

Dicky's voice sounded from the opposite side of the room. A hand waved and I pushed a way through the omnipresent khaki throng to join him. Spilled one man's drink on the way, but he appeared too drunk to notice.

'Dicky, how you doing?'

'Grand, grand. Here you go, mate.' A beer was handed over. 'Be with you in a moment.' He turned back to his group. 'Anyway, this naked woman's running through the forest. The gamekeeper sees her, thinks to himself 'aye, aye' and sets off in pursuit. Chases her for hours he does.' Dicky allowed himself a chuckle, 'Finally catches her. She turns around and she's gorgeous, lads. He says "Are you game?" She says "Oh yes." So he shot her!'

Dicky roared with laughter and his companions copied. It was hard to tell how many people were with him, the room so packed with bodies. Three women sat at a nearby table and I wondered if the nurse he'd mentioned could be one of these.

I ordered another Blue Label, the first one swallowed quickly. I felt nervous to meet a new crowd, and definitely reluctant to be set up.

'All right, Harry!' Dicky turned to face me, his usual slap on the back. 'Sorry about that. Telling the lads some jokes, got to keep them happy, eh? So how's life at the hospital, then?'

'Boring me to tears, Dicky. I've been looking forward to this all week.'

'Well I'd better tell you who's who then. Going to be a long night.'

He shouted names and faces nodded back, but only one is now remembered.

Nan.

She sat in front of me, around the table. I had guessed right. Nan wore a white blouse and the first thing to catch my eye, if I'm honest, was the fine gold chain plunging down between her breasts. My gaze was quick to lift higher.

She was beautiful. Dark velvet hair flowed to her shoulders, brushed out of her face with long, elegant fingers. This framed a lovely, olive complexion and I found myself drawn into her brown eyes. They shone so deep and clear, pure as moonlight, and I wanted to dive into their oceans. To be carried far away, helpless, wherever they took me. She smiled often, a good smile, not only with her mouth but using her entire face.

Dicky's whisper broke my reverie. 'So you like her then?' I nodded.

'Remember Harry, things are different out here. It's another world. Don't let the past get in the way.'

Her lips were full, always a good sign, her nose petite. From where I stood, the buttons of Nan's blouse breathed open to allow sight of a delicate white strap of underclothing, caressing the dark skin of her shoulder. I couldn't stop myself from looking at it.

One of her friends, laughing, knocked a box of matches onto the floor. Nan bent to retrieve this and her blouse breathed open further. I now glimpsed a birthmark, deep red, at the top of her chest. I'd never seen anything as lovely.

It took another beer and several more of Dicky's bad jokes before I'd finally relaxed. Still we hadn't spoken. It was Nan who stood suddenly, her movements fluid as a dancer, and she walked towards me as slowly and inevitable as an incoming tide.

'Hello Harry, I'm Nan.'

She bent forwards to kiss me on the cheek, one arm about my shoulders. Amazed, I stood stiffly, feeling both clumsy and awkward.

'Hello Nan. How do you know Dicky?'

'I don't really.' Her smile was even better close up. I detected a faint scent of perfume, white musk. 'He knows my friends. And you?'

'We come from the same town back in England, Folkestone. Didn't expect to see him out here.'

Nan continued to maintain eye contact, continued to smile, and butterflies danced swift pirouettes in my stomach. 'Where are you from?' I asked.

'Marsaxlokk. It's a small fishing village on the east coast. So how do you like Malta?' The voice was warm, honest.

'It's been good so far, but I've not been here long. Only really seen Sliema and Valletta, and thankfully not much action. What's it like in - where was it - Marsaxlokk?'

She touched my arm, gently correcting the pronunciation, and I felt immense disappointment when she withdrew her hand. I was as giddy as a schoolboy.

'It's nice. Not very big, but pretty. Of course it's a little different now, with everything else, but I still like it. You should come and visit.'

'I'd love that. Would you take me?'

'Maybe.' She touched my arm, again. 'So you're another nurse, do you like this work?'

'I loved it back home. Don't really know what to expect out here. Dicky said you're a nurse, too. Whereabouts?'

'I'm in Valletta, the surgical wards. It's okay at the moment, but it was terrible a few months back. I preferred it before the war, of course.'

'You must have had some casualties.' I'd heard about the attacks on *Illustrious* when she was moored in the harbour. 'How do you prepare for that?'

Nan shook her head, sadly, and I cursed myself for removing her smile.

'You can't. It's impossible.' She paused. 'So tell me about Folkestone. Is it near London?'

'Not that near. Actually, I live in London, but I still go home to see the parents.'

'This is good, Harry' the smile returned. 'I think the family is very important.'

'Me too, Nan.' I exaggerated my opinion, happy to agree with her. 'Folkestone is quite small, but it's on the coast. Got a lovely old harbour where I learned to swim.'

'I love swimming! I love the sea. We also have a harbour in Marsaxlokk.'

'Well, that's another thing we have in common, then.'

I spotted Dicky's wink and turned away. He wasn't going to put me off tonight. I knew immediately that Nan was a good, kind, woman. She was obviously intelligent, of strong opinions, which I liked. Her laughter arrived in explosions, as if she herself was surprised by it. Nan's whole body shook, and I shook with her. When she wound a finger, thoughtful, into her hair, I found myself attracted with a passion I had never known. When she gazed down at her own shapely legs, I was smitten.

I wondered how this could be possible. It could have been due to the way she shared details of her life, already intimate, the frequent touches on my arm. It could have been the way she listened, turning her body to face me, her head bent slightly to one side. Her dark eyes were just incredible.

My gaze kept returning to the white strap on her shoulder. I felt jealous that it was not my finger, my lips. I would have no choice in this; I felt drawn to Nan with forces beyond my control. When I made her laugh, I knew then that love had found me. There could be no other explanation.

We managed to slip unnoticed from the bar, at her suggestion.

'Quick, Harry, before they spot us. There's something you must see.'

She took my hand as if it was the most natural act in the world. My heart raced so fast, I was sure that Nan would notice. We turned left onto Kingsway, where all was quiet. Walking down shallow stone steps towards the Fort, the streets were totally deserted.

'Where are we going, Nan?' I spoke softly, not wishing to disturb this calm.

'You'll see.' She squeezed my hand. 'Not far.'

Fort St. Elmo loomed out of the darkness, threatening, and I was glad to be on the right side of it. The thick stone walls appeared impossible to breach, enlarged by the ghostly light. No wonder the Italians had failed in their attack.

We turned left again. Fountain Street. Nan quickened her stride, pulling me across the road.

'Look, Harry! What do you think?'

A cool breeze blanketed us, so welcome after the bar. Bright stars pierced the ink blue sky. Across the harbour towards Sliema, the sea shimmered pearly with moonlight.

'It's beautiful, Nan.'

'I know! That's why I brought you here. It looks even better at night.' She looked upwards, 'And no raids tonight. It's perfect.'

She rested her head against my shoulder, I wrapped my arm around her. It was the first time that I'd felt completely at ease with another person. I believed that I could tell Nan anything. That she would listen, and understand me.

The night whispered sweet nothings. We continued our walk, slowly now, without words. St. Sebastian Street. I was aware of Nan slowing further, and only then noticed the gunpost in front of us. This had to be avoided; we needed to keep the war at bay, at least for a little longer.

'Come on, Nan. Follow me,' I whispered.

'Where?'

'My turn to take you somewhere. A surprise.'

I'd spotted three arches on the opposite side of the road, and now I was the one leading. Beneath the third arch, an entrance to a tiny street, we turned as one. Moonlight and shadow danced across her features. I placed a hand gently onto Nan's face, stroking her cheek.

'You,' she whispered.

I held her against me and we kissed. The first time.

'Are you always like this, Harry?'

'How do you mean?'

We still held onto each other.

'Tonight. The men who approached me before were more forward, cruder. It makes a nice change.'

'I'm a gentleman, Nan. There's not many of us left.'

She smiled at me. 'Good. Have you ever been different?'

'Not really. No.' I couldn't bring myself to mention Gwen's name, my previous life in London.

'Your bristles are probably giving me a rash.'

'It's the heat, I think, making them grow faster. Sorry, I'll sort it out.'

'Next time?'

'Yes.'

She bent towards me and we kissed again.

'So when can I see you again, Nan?'

'Can't make tomorrow, it's Sunday. What about Monday afternoon? I finish early.'

'You're on. Where?'

'Fountain Street, near the Fort.'

CHAPTER FIVE

My eyelids felt heavy, reluctant to open. It was a struggle to raise myself, squinting at my watch in the darkness of the room, and I scowled – I could have slept for longer, another hour at least. But then my thoughts returned to yesterday, and to Nan.

I couldn't wait to see her in M'tarfa. I wanted to kiss her again, to stroke the curves of her body, to watch her undress. That birthmark alone drove me crazy with desire - it looked so damn beautiful. Her hair, eyes, smell, personality; I loved it all. Everything. She was perfect, a miracle that I'd found her.

Balling the palms of my hands firmly against both eyelids, attempting to get up, all I could see was Nan. Dark eyes, full lips, her smile. I flopped back onto the pillow, a happy man.

Cleaning my teeth, I was aware that something hurt inside my mouth. Closer inspection revealed a small bite-mark on the underside of my tongue. Caused by Nan. I felt proud, suddenly ecstatic. I hoped it would never heal. After bundling my gear into a bag, it was then a race to the collection point. An Austin utility van soon arrived and the driver was expecting me. The sun already boiled in the sky, the light dazzling. Quickly, we left Sliema and the hospital.

I was surprised how green the land became once we'd departed from the coast. Both our windows were open, and beautiful perfumes scented the warm air. We bumped past old farmhouses and stone walls that had obviously baked undisturbed in the sunshine for many years. There were countless fields of potatoes, with mustard yellow Cape

Sorrel adding a pleasant contrast to surroundings. The driver spoke little, and this suited me fine. I was content just to think about Nan.

Moving further inland, the country again became barren. The dusty fields here were empty of crops, the dry land unforgiving. I felt my stomach tense with worry, but the driver merely shrugged. 'There's a war on,' he said.

Half-hour later, I was deposited at the barracks in M'tarfa. This was a small town of angular Moorish houses, with army quarters located on the outskirts. The barracks comprised a row of modest grey two-storey blocks. They were oblong, plain in appearance, not ugly, and would now have to be home.

I was directed to my room by the driver - under the arch, up six steps, first door on the left. Four almond trees stood outside the building, the stone radiating a faint orange light. Sweet birdsong graced the air and I bounded inside, keen to investigate.

The room was found at the end of the block. Inside it was cool and dark, three tiny slits in the stone an excuse for a window. The furniture comprised an iron camp bed and adjacent wooden cabinet, nothing else. It smelled of stale sweat and Brylcreem. I wondered what had happened to the previous occupant, whether he was now one of the casualties. It was a small, depressing space, but I unpacked immediately, trying to make it feel more comfortable. Love and war spun my world faster than ever, and I was determined to hold on tightly.

It was a five minute walk, straight down St. David's Road and its muddle of houses, to reach the hospital. When I first saw this building, hiding behind ancient olive trees, I was surprised by the size. M'tarfa hospital was an impressive three-storey affair of thick yellow stone, reminiscent of an English stately home. I felt glad to join its staff, particularly after the experience of Sliema.

A wide drive meandered through colourful gardens to reach the main entrance, and I stopped to admire burning bright red hibiscus plants, their buds rolled tightly into little fists. Oleander trees were plentiful, abundant with red and white flowers, together with almond and fig trees. It was quiet, definitely a place to allow healing.

The same green shutters covered the windows that I'd noticed often in Valletta, with shaded balconies visible on every level of the building. Even the roof was adorned with fancy stonework. But when I walked up the driveway, the hospital suddenly looked like the saddest building I'd ever seen. I thought I could sense ghosts of the dead searching lost along the long, cool, corridors. Young men, who'd once been like me, stranded a long way from home. It was the same from every angle, an overpowering sensation, and yet death was never an option in my own mind. I knew that Nan was on her way.

I meandered past a large red cross painted within the grounds and this puzzled me at first. But then I realised its purpose, to be visible from the air. A small chapel was found to the right of the building, dedicated to St. Oswald. It was surprisingly ornate, surrounded by pale sandstone columns, and complete with its own little dome. I lent against a column, took a deep breath, brushed down my uniform, then walked beyond this and into the hospital reception.

'Harold Fisher. Reporting for duty.'

A tiny Maltese lady gazed at me quizzically from behind a desk situated near to the door. She was dark-skinned and plump, similar to most of the older women I had met.

'I've been sent from Sliema.'

'Oh yes.' A flicker of recollection, a smile. 'We've been expecting you. Welcome. Welcome. Come in. I'll get Matron.'

She offered me her chair and dashed away, retreating along a straight corridor that led into the heart of the building. I chose to stand. The hospital appeared to be spotlessly clean, smarting with a strong smell of familiar disinfectant. Inside, all was silent.

'Fisher?' A figure appeared in the distance, emerging from a doorway halfway along the corridor.

'That's right.'

'You've made it then, good.' She walked towards me. 'We can always use another pair of hands. I've told Sister McHardy to show you around. She's on her way now. I'm the matron.' She offered her hand, a vice-like grip.

Matron was English, a trim, efficient-looking lady of indeterminate age. Her brown hair was tied back severely, lending an appearance of mild surprise. There was a formidable quality about her; I could never imagine her as a child or younger woman. She wore a sharply pressed white dress and studied me closely through large oval spectacles. I struggled to find my voice. She made me nervous.

'Harold Fisher. It's good to be here.'

'Well, I hope you're saying that tomorrow. We run a tight ship. Here comes Sister McHardy, now.' I turned to the door, where a smiling young lady with strawberry-blonde hair stood waiting. 'You'll be taking over from her. Well, I must get back to my duties. I'm sure I'll be seeing you later.'

Matron spun sharply and strode purposefully away. She appeared to float, making no sound at all on the hard stone floor.

'Sister McHardy?'

'Yes, that's me. Are you Harold?' She spoke with a broad Scottish accent, reminding me of Kerr.

'I am.'

'Well pleased to meet you, then. And do call me Anna. I'm glad I found you. Matron's always in such a hurry, she didn't tell me where you'd be.'

Anna was tall and slim, her pale complexion spotted with widening freckles. She spoke incredibly quickly.

'So you're my replacement, eh? I'll be sorry to go. They're sending me to Egypt - supposed to be safer, but I'd have been just as happy staying. Well come on then, the tour starts here. Where are you from Harold?'

'Sliema. Not been here long.'

'No, silly,' she laughed, throaty with good humour. 'I meant back home, England.'

'London,' I smiled, 'but originally from Folkestone. What about you?'

'Aberdeen. I miss the old place, and the weather. Too warm for me here. Well come on with you then, better get moving.'

The main hospital building was well designed with large airy wards, apparently far superior to the one at Sliema. It was cool, well ventilated, and each ward appeared to be immaculate. I'd expected more basic conditions and admitted this to Anna.

'Well we've no choice really, Harold,' she laughed. 'That wee Matron is always checking up on us. You don't want to go crossing her, no way. If you only remember one thing today, that's it!'

We had reached the end of the corridor. An open window looked out onto more gardens at the rear of the building, where a prickly pear tapped gently against the wooden frame.

'Harold, you've got to see this.' Anna began to climb the staircase on our left. 'You won't believe it.'

She set a brisk pace, pausing only once to allow me to catch up.

'Always a breeze out here, Harold, if you ever need to cool down.'

'So where are we going, Anna?'

'The roof, of course. You want to see the view!'

We emerged into bright white sunlight. The hospital stood on high ground, its size providing a grandstand view of the island.

'We're standing on top of the operating theatre right now, so we are.' Anna giggled. 'Have to tiptoe, don't want to disturb them. So what do you think?'

I scanned the horizon, turning slowly. A ribbon of blue confirmed that the sea would never be far away, and I could make out an airfield in front of this. The barrack blocks were clearly visible, and beyond these an old fortified town rose vertically from the dry earth.

'It's fantastic, Anna. So where's that?'

'Mdina. They call it the silent city. You'll have to visit there Harold, I love it. It's my favourite place on the island, to get away from it all. A bit different from home, eh?'

It was a sticky, sweaty heat. The wind scorched hot on my face, all clouds shaken clear from the sky.

'You're right. But over there, that reminds me of St. Paul's.' I pointed left of the airfield, towards a large church.

'Aye. It's Mosta Cathedral, third largest dome in Europe, so I'm told.'

'Where's Valletta, Anna?'

'Well you can't really see it, but it would be that way.'

She pointed in a direction between the airfield and Mosta. 'Only time it's obvious is when it's under attack. You'll see the smoke clearly then, right enough.'

'It's great up here, Anna, thanks.'

'Well, I'd better take you back down now, or we'll have Matron on our backs. You don't want that on your first day, I can tell you!'

'Where's Marsaxlokk, quickly?'

'I don't know that one, Harold. Probably too far away.'

We returned down the stairs and into the gardens. Anna walked towards several barrack blocks that she told me had recently been converted into extra medical wards.

'This is it, Harold.' We stood outside one of the buildings. 'Only problem with this place, it's not big enough.'

'But it looks massive, Anna,' I protested.

'Sorry, Harold, but it's not big enough for what they're expecting. Had to expand, and fast. Know what it reminds me of out here? Cardboard boxes! All been done on the cheap of course, too quickly, but that's no surprise. Harold, you'll be based here. F Block,' she read the sign. 'Welcome to your new home!'

Several unoccupied beds had been positioned outside, in the shade. F Block had an upstairs and downstairs balcony. It looked a considerable size.

'Come in then, Harold.' She pushed open the door. 'One hundred beds, for infectious diseases. I'll tell you all you need to know.'

The ward stood empty, a skeleton waiting for flesh. It was refreshingly cool, and I spotted that all the windows had been fitted with fine mesh to keep the insects out. The beds were already in line, a second mattress lying underneath each frame. It stank of carbolic acid, and Anna noticed me wince.

'What is it, Harold? Cold feet?'

'No, not at all. It's that smell. Horrible.'

'Ach that's nothing' she laughed, 'you soon get used to it. I'd forgotten it was there. Anyway, if things get too bad it'll soon run out. You'll be using water after that.'

'Is it really so important, Anna?'

'Afraid so. You'll see. These buildings are all infested with bugs. It's an ongoing battle, but you'll get used to it, right enough. They're old, not ideal for a hospital, but we have to make do. Come in.' She walked towards a desk at the far end of the ward. 'I'd better show you the paperwork. Matron's always a stickler for that.'

It was a long day, with much to learn, but Anna remained patient throughout. She was an excellent teacher and pleasant company with it.

'I'm sorry you have to go,' I admitted.

'Ach, Harold, you'll soon have picked it up. Don't fret yourself.'

'But I would have liked to work with you. You're obviously good at the job.'

Anna possessed that ability to communicate, to spread calm, so important in nursing.

'Are you making a move, you wee charmer? Didn't take you long, did it!' She roared with laughter.

'No,' I laughed with her. 'I meant just what I said.'

The sun sank gently out of the sky, bestowing a warm orange sheen to the day. I returned to barracks for a plate of bangers and mash in the Mess and then it was back to my room. There was a lot to take in, with little time before Anna departed for Egypt.

The air in the room was stale. I undressed, sweating, and

flopped wearily onto the bed. Closing my eyes, countless images of Nan swam before me, automatically projected onto the backs of my eyelids like the flicking of a switch. She was in the Union Jack, on Fountain Street, her bedroom. She was smiling, looking straight at me. I was so impatient for her. Sleep was again slow to arrive.

In the morning, it was an early start on F Block. Anna waited for me, and I was allocated a small Maltese staff to help with the nursing. To my relief, they all spoke excellent English. Anna provided them with their instruction.

'Your hours will be alternate shifts of 8 a.m. until 1 p.m. and 8 a.m. until 8 p.m. There'll be one free day per week. We'll start receiving patients later this week, so our first job is the cleaning. Matron will be along to check soon, so we'd better have everything spotless. Any questions?'

There were none, and the staff set purposefully about their work.

'You'll see they're good, Harold,' Anna whispered. 'Won't give you any problems.'

'I'm still sorry you're leaving.'

She smiled, her cheeks creased with deep laughter lines. 'Well I can help you this week, when we get some patients. Should all be pretty routine, but there'll be a few things you haven't seen before. You'll soon pick it up, like I said. It was just the same for me when I got here.'

Our day was spent disinfecting the mattresses and greasing bed frames, as I'd done in Sliema. Small tins were again positioned under the iron legs, and again these required repeated topping up. Sweating profusely, cursing, I was not happy. Anna noticed this and walked over, chuckling.

'Remember to delegate, once the admissions start,' she whispered.

On the third day in M'tarfa, Anna went through specific protocols for the duties that I'd be expected to perform. There were sheets of written instructions detailing the nursing of various dysenteries and diarrhoeas, the usual source of admissions. One disease I'd never heard of was Undulant Fever, which she assured me was dying out. It was contracted almost exclusively from drinking infected goat milk. There was a scheme for pasteurisation now in place, but sometimes the local farmers persisted in bringing their animals directly to the customer's door.

Protocols were also in place detailing the event of an air raid. I knew already about the purpose of the second mattress, but those patients who were mobile were expected to shelter in slit trenches, outside. Anna showed me where these were located, deep scars cut into the rocky ground about the hospital.

'What about the Red Cross? Doesn't that make any difference?' I enquired.

She smiled kindly, suppressing a laugh.

'No difference, Harold. Doesn't count for anything.' Anna hesitated, unfamiliar anger suddenly infecting her voice. 'I'm sure some of the cheeky wee shites aim for it!'

There had been a period of relative quiet since my arrival on the island. German planes were thankfully scarce, and it was the Italians who remained responsible for sporadic raids. This wasn't as bad; they didn't come in close like the Germans, preferring the safer, less accurate, option of bombing from great height.

The hospital roof was the ideal place to view proceedings, and Anna had already directed me to the best vantage point.

Groups of men were always assembled above the operating theatre, and here we could watch planes become visible as tiny pinheads in the distance, a darkening cloud on the horizon. When they grew closer, slowly enlarging, it was possible to hear the monotonous drone of the engines.

We watched the moment of release, bombs glinting, twinkling, and sparkling, against a perfect azure sky. They resembled treasure on a seabed, or Christmas baubles, nothing remotely in their appearance to suggest imminent death and destruction. Sometimes, it was possible to identify white puffs of anti-aircraft fire.

The view of Mosta Cathedral continued to remind me of London. My previous life began to float back to me, like a long forgotten story, much as I tried to forget it. But since arriving in M'tarfa, there had been no news heard from Nan. I was haunted by her face in every woman that I saw, always checking for identification, for recognition. Every time, I was disappointed. It was never her.

I still remembered the silk curve of her neck when she smiled, the way she tidied hair behind her ear using two fingers. I pictured the silver ring on her right hand, its cut out shapes and patterns. I recalled the way she had stood at Fountain Street, one leg bent slightly in front of the other. I loved to imagine the flick of her dark hair on a pillow, and over me. I could never grow bored of reliving our first kiss. Doubts began to throw shapes in my mind. What if she wouldn't get here, after all? If she'd had a change of heart? We hadn't much time for things to develop between us, what if I'd been mistaken, if I had misread the situation? I could not stop it, my thoughts finally returned to London. And to Gwen.

CHAPTER SIX

I arrived in London in 1935, filled with excitement and high hopes to commence training as a State Registered Nurse. My previous employees, the Reverend Joseph Hocking and his kind wife, had provided the necessary encouragement, reference, and financial support, with the result that I'd been offered a place at the National Hospital for Diseases of the Nervous System.

The train from Folkestone terminated at Charing Cross Station, and I treated myself to a taxi cab. After my home town, London seemed to go on forever, a seabed of ever-changing buildings and green parkland. I felt an awed reverence at the numbers of people, the tremendous size of the place.

The driver dropped me off at Guilford Street, directing me into a lovely, airy square for the hospital. Suddenly, the wind blew up a gale from out of nowhere and the rain came horizontal. I'd made an effort to be smart for the day, to set a good impression, and now it would all be ruined. I could feel my new trousers stick damp onto the backs of my legs. My hair was plastered untidily across my face.

I jogged to the right side of the square, wondering which building could be the hospital. It wasn't the one I'd aimed for. A man rushed past, umbrella in hand, and I tried to catch his attention but he ignored me. That would never have happened in Folkestone.

I stood still, forcing myself to calm down, to think. A public garden was in the middle of the square, the statue of a lonely woman visible rising above the tree line. Beyond this, I could now see a handsome, red-brick building of tidy size. It looked grand enough to be a National Hospital and I ran straight into the garden, hoping to discover a shortcut.

The rain continued to smack against me. I was getting wetter and wetter, a drowned appearance, but when the path led directly to the statue I stopped and stared. I looked up at her face, the funeral murk of the sky, and watched a single tear of rain roll down her cheek. I ran on.

The building was indeed the National, thank goodness. Reception was located to the right of the entrance hall, vivid stained glass windows above the staircase in front of me. There was nobody at the desk so I pressed once on the shiny brass bell.

A young man, already bald, appeared from a back room. He looked me up and down before speaking in what I assumed to be a London accent.

'Raining, is it?'

I explained who I was and he smiled.

'Okay mate, I'll get you Sister Elliott.'

Sister Elliott was quick to appear, a middle-aged redhead of slight build. She had a kind smile and shook my hand with genuine warmth.

'Welcome to the National, Harold. You've certainly picked a good day to arrive.'

I must have looked a sight, dripping copious amounts of rainwater onto the clean tiles of the floor. I made an attempt to smooth back my hair.

'I'll show you to your lodgings, and give you a quick look around the place on the way. Your room will be on Guilford Street, but we don't need to get ourselves wet.'

She led me down a staircase where we entered a subterranean labyrinth of winding passages and courtyards. Here, the fogged, green light of the corridor felt like diving beneath the sea.

'Better tell you some of the rules. You've done well to get a place here Harold, don't want to let yourself down now. We're known all over the world, and expect high standards.'

She walked quickly, and I hurried to keep behind her.

'It's never allowed to run inside these corridors,' she turned to check I was listening. 'If somebody senior approaches, you must always step aside to let them pass. Ward duties start at seven punctually, but there'll be a wake up call at six.'

We came to the end of the passage and began to climb another staircase.

'Guilford Street, Harold. It's joined to the hospital, no need to go outside. We're in the basement, but you'll be staying on the third floor. I'll show you to your room, and then you can meet me back at reception in thirty minutes. I'll take you around the hospital wards.'

The room was large, with four beds. I had a private locker, but would have to share the wardrobe and chest of drawers. This wasn't a problem as I didn't carry many belongings. Outside, a tree blocked the light through our window.

I threw my bag onto the one empty bed. Clean sheets were folded, ready for use, and I used the pillowcase to towel myself down. Dot's bear was placed carefully into the locker, and I returned to the hospital reception. Unpacking could wait until later.

Sister Elliott guided me through various wards and departments. The hospital amazed me, filled with beautiful pictures, stained glass, and dayrooms. It even had a good-sized library. I was introduced to a sea of smiling faces and began to wonder how I'd remember anything.

'Don't worry, Harold,' she must have read my thoughts,

'I'll be around to help.'

We worked long hours on those wards, and lectures were scheduled during off-duty periods. It was certainly hard work, but after the year I'd spent unemployed, visiting the dreaded Labour Exchange, I was glad of this. My roommates were a decent bunch of lads and I quickly settled into a routine.

Night duties were the hardest. Fourteen consecutive shifts had to be completed before gaining two free days. Sometimes you were lucky, and the hours passed quickly in study. That was when patients remained sleeping and comfortable, but epileptic fits were a common event in a neurological hospital. Catching people as they fell, keeping them free from injury, could be difficult physical work. I once had two fingers bitten to the bone when attempting to clear the airway of a young male patient, leaving me with scars that resembled flashes of lightning. Another time, to the delight of my friends, I was struck viciously on the back of the head by a patient wielding a urine bottle. It took months to live that episode down, even Sister Elliott having a laugh at my expense. All this, and it was necessary to prepare and eat your own meals on the ward.

When I needed some quiet, I visited the chapel on the ground floor. I would always sit near to the back, running my eyes slowly over the mosaic floor. Silence washed through the room. Black, yellow, white, brown tiles; I thought of all the patients I'd looked after, hoping they were doing all right, that there had been no mistakes in the nursing. Here, I found gazing at the stained glass windows to be calming.

Shortage of funds proved the biggest problem during that first year. On a miserly salary of twenty five pounds per annum, I was particularly grateful for the money that the

Hockings had provided. Mum also helped out, often posting a ten-shilling note sewn carefully into the pages of the Folkestone Herald newspaper to avoid detection. With these extras, I made sure that I found time for the exploration of London.

I had kept in touch with Dot Golding, through occasional letters. She'd told me about her current boyfriend and apparently it was serious. I could accept and cope with this, still grateful for the time we had once enjoyed, and it was Dot who introduced me to the man who became my closest friend.

Six feet tall, fourteen stone of lean, compact muscle, I was initially in awe of Eric Reynolds. His perfect teeth were set in a strong jaw, above this startling green eyes, a full head of immaculate greased black hair. He was everything that I wanted to be, and for a long time I felt unsure why he should accept me as his companion.

Eric also came from Folkestone, although we'd never met, and now worked as assistant casting director for a Soho-based stage and film agency. I couldn't imagine a more glamorous vocation, and his movie star good looks often earned him parts as a film extra. I could not have wished for a better friend.

He always seemed to be in possession of complimentary tickets. We visited the theatres around Piccadilly Circus, watched musicals on Shaftsbury Avenue that moved me for days afterwards, and cheered on the Gunners at Highbury whenever possible. This London life seemed impossibly exciting after a relatively quiet upbringing on the coast. And it got even better, too. When Eric paired up with a stunner on our jaunts about the city, I invariably ended up with her friend, the cheerful good sport.

He took everything that life threw at him with calmness, apparently unflappable, and I might have felt resentment, or even envy, had he not been such a kind, generous man. Eric laughed as if he meant it with every ounce of his being, possessing the deep, guttural roar of a sea lion. His company was both a delight and a privilege; he was a great person to show me the city.

We once appeared together in a movie, sitting as extras on the top deck of a bus that trundled up and down Acton Road. The stars were John Loder and the beautiful American Sylvia Sidney. She shot us a sultry 'Thank you boys' when making her departure, and I received a magnificent two guineas for my time.

Our finest night would have to be the Chelsea Arts Ball held in the Royal Albert Hall. I'd seen brief clips of this event in the cinemas back home, never once imagining that I should attend. Typical of Eric, he managed to obtain the ticket, dinner jacket, and even my date for the night. I had never felt so grand or witnessed such glamour. Real pearls and diamonds glistened like stars plucked down from the sky. I danced the night away in a dream world of champagne and sparkling, twinkling lights.

Life at the hospital continued to agree with me. The rules were strict and ward duties demanding, but I would not allow myself to become unemployed again. Several colleagues resigned, or were forced to quit through ill health. One of my roommates died, a nasty bout of diphtheria, but I pushed myself to work harder and harder.

The training grew in both interest and enjoyment. I spent seven months on placement in the operating theatre, the National at the forefront of pioneering new techniques. Neurosurgery usually took between three to four hours, and

I sometimes worked a fifteen-hour day. It was important to remain physically fit.

The first operation in which I assisted was on a Saturday afternoon. A Cockney lad, twelve years old, was admitted in emergency suffering from a suspected acute cerebral abscess. Success being critical on time, it was my job to hold him still while the local anaesthetic was injected directly into his scalp. I watched the patient's hair rise up and, after a brief wait, the surgeon commenced drilling.

This produced a terrible grinding sound, but it was nothing compared to the animal screams of that boy. I pressed thick towels over his ears, to muffle the noise of the drill, but he continued to kick and fight. It smelt dreadful, burning, as his temporal bone was carefully peeled away to create access into the brain.

A hole was eventually opened, and the abscess burst with an audible pop. Thick yellow fluid was drained from the wound, later healing uneventful. In recovery, the boy admitted how he'd been more frightened than hurt, but I never became used to the screams of children. It was at this time that training included lumbar puncture and the operation of an iron lung.

1936 arrived at speed, the year the King abdicated and gave up everything for love. It was the year that spawned the Spanish Civil War. Eric and I had discovered a decent café run by two confirmed Socialists, Overton and Hadley. It was basic, a little dirty, but there was an inviting Bohemian feel to the place. Brightly painted slogans written in Spanish were daubed onto the walls. The food was cheap and good.

Hadley had recently lost a brother who was fighting in the International Brigade against Franco, and these two earnest men took it as their duty to educate Eric and me. In

Spain, civilian populations were being deliberately bombed for the first time. When they explained the political ideal behind this war, it sounded tremendously exciting and worthy. We listened spellbound, over countless smokes, when they argued with one of Sir Oswald Mosley's black-shirted recruits. War was made to sound an attractive proposition, and I was quickly hooked. We stayed out so late that I often had to sneak back into my Guilford Street lodgings through a ground floor window - it could result in instant dismissal if caught outside out of hours.

1936 was important for another reason. Eric invited me out for a drink with his friend Elsie Galey. He often spoke of her in glowing terms, but our paths had never crossed. I was definitely keen to meet her.

In a Shepherd's Bush pub, Eric made the usual introductions and I was surprised to find that Elsie was plain in appearance; this was most unusual among his female friends. A mass of frizzy brown hair, squinting eyes magnified through milk-bottle lenses, I quickly discovered that she possessed a fantastic sense of humour. But it was the other member of our party who immediately caught my eye.

Gwendoline Sylvia Fletcher, she said to call her Gwen, appeared cultured, distant, and bore a striking resemblance to the actress Greta Garbo. This was enhanced through emulation of Garbo's hair, make-up, and even mannerisms. Everybody in London seemed to be falling in love and there was a quality of sadness, of vulnerability, about Gwen, that I found tremendously attractive. She wore a pale blue blouse and slim fitting black trousers. Gwen turned away whenever I studied her, apparently distracted by a commotion in the doorway, but I detected her own gaze on me when she thought I was chatting to Eric.

As the evening danced past, I noticed how Gwen even spoke like Garbo, in clipped, measured tones. I'd never met anyone like this - we did not get such women back in Folkestone. She appeared more interested in me than Eric, which was again definitely unusual. I learned that she hailed from Brixton, and had trained with Elsie at both the Fountain and Oldchurch Hospitals. She was currently employed as a nurse in the psychiatric unit of the Central Middlesex Hospital.

We decided to continue the party at Gwen's Uxbridge Road flat. She leaned heavily against me as we stood to leave the pub, linking arms, and I was briefly aware of the weight of her breasts pressing onto my arm.

The flat turned out to be a modest affair, situated on the second floor of a row of terraced houses. It consisted of two main rooms, a bedroom and living room. The kitchen and bathroom were enclosed in a separate annex reached from the hallway. It was sparsely furnished, but scrupulously clean and tidy.

A bottle of brandy was produced from Eric's coat like a rabbit pulled out of a hat, and glasses quickly found in the kitchen. Here, a picture of a rainbow was stuck onto one of the walls. Eric and Elsie were deep in conversation when Gwen beckoned in my direction.

'Come here, Harold. There's something I want to show you.'

Right from the beginning, she never once called me Harry. She offered a cold hand and led me into the hall. Gwen opened the nearest window.

'Just climb outside.'

'What's out there, Gwen?'

'You'll see.'

I followed her command to find myself standing above the ground floor bay window, where Gwen had positioned a small wooden bench. I shuffled along while she climbed nimbly out to join me, and we sat side-by-side watching the sky become heavy with stars. Night buses trundled past at regular intervals. The cool air hissed static. We were not quite touching.

'I don't know why Harold, but you make me want to tell you about myself.' Gwen spoke more quietly now, her accent disappeared. 'That doesn't happen often. Do you believe in happiness?' She glanced at me quickly, then back to the sky. 'I don't think I'll ever be happy.'

'But why?' I'd never been asked or considered such a question. I knew I wanted to be of help.

'I just know it. My background's partly to do with it.' She glanced again in my direction. 'Can I talk to you?'

'Of course. Yes.' Gwen held me captive. She excited, delighted, and frightened me, all at the same time. She continued to speak, her voice now halting and weak.

'My mother died giving birth to me, not the best start in life. I felt cursed and father didn't help at all, shipping me off as soon as possible to live with a grandmother. She was a loveable old dear, but then she went and died too. It's stupid, I know, but as a girl I couldn't help thinking it must be my fault.'

'Poor you.' I inched closer to her side.

'Anyway, father remarried. Miss Ruby Lloyd.' She spat this name out, a first glimpse of venom. 'He met her when he was in the navy. She was a concert singer, and couldn't stand children. She made sure I had an unhappy time of it. Of course, she then went and got pregnant. But lost it. She chose to blame me, saying I made an unhappy atmosphere in the house. You can't do that to a child, can you Harold?'

'No. She sounds horrible.'

'She was a bitch.' Gwen paused, as if surprised by the strength of her words. 'I was sent packing again, this time to a friend of theirs. I'd even won a scholarship Harold, but she wouldn't let me take it. I was sent to be their domestic.'

I took gentle hold of her arm and was pleased when she made no attempt to move away. Again, I inched closer.

'They worked me so hard. I never saw father and I had to get out. To escape. That's when I applied to the Fountain Hospital and met Elsie.' Gwen smiled now. 'She's such a love. We worked together on the children's ward and qualified together. I told you that, in the pub. I even began to see father again. I think he was proud of his girl, and he came to my graduation. But then it went really wrong, Harold.'

Gwen suddenly burst into tears, a pained sobbing that sent deep shudders throughout her body. I wrapped my arm around her, pulling her close, feeling out of my depth and lost at sea.

'What happened?'

'I met a man, Clem. We fell in love. You know how it is.'

I did not. It seemed I was learning fast.

'We married, and straight away I became pregnant. Clem then left me, the bastard, for another woman. Father had warned that he was a bad choice, and now he refused to help. He disowned me! Miss Lloyd made him, I know. Everyone leaves me Harold, sooner or later.'

Gwen continued to cry. I didn't know what to say and attempted to hug her. She was rigid in my arms, but again I could feel the weight of her breasts pressing against me. She turned, her eyes empty of expression. My discomfort grew steadily until a small smile forced itself onto her face.

'I had the child, Harold. Diana. She's just turned one and friends take care of her for me, in Essex. She's a lovely little thing. That's why I came to the Middlesex. I like it there. I like it here.'

I continued to hold Gwen, afraid to let go. Her last words clung to the air, rich with promise. We both gazed up at the stars, finally able to enjoy the night silence.

'It's getting cold,' Gwen spoke abruptly. 'I'm going inside.'

I sat on my own. It had been quite a night - it always was with Eric, but Gwen was something else. I felt torn with conflicting emotions for this incredible woman, of pity, and also desire. All things considered, I thought it might be more sensible to make my excuses and leave for Guilford Street.

Climbing through the window, back into the flat, Eric and Elsie had disappeared. They had already gone home. I walked into the living room to collect my jacket and say goodbye, and it was then that I noticed the strip of light visible beneath the bedroom door. It reeled me in slowly, reluctantly, trapped like a fish on a line.

The door was slightly ajar, with no sounds heard from within. I stood motionless, indecisive, before plucking up courage and pushing it gently open.

She was standing in front of the dressing table, wearing a fitted black basque and French-style knickers. Her right foot was positioned on a small red velvet stool. Gwen very slowly unrolled a black silk stocking to reveal immaculate porcelain white flesh. I could not move. She must have known that I was there for she looked up and held my gaze. She then returned to her task until one stocking had been removed.

Her leg looked perfect. I wanted to reach in, to touch, but stood rooted to the spot. Slowly, deliberately, Gwen swapped legs in order that her left foot now rested on the stool. For one long moment in time, delicious and slow, she again rolled the stocking down until it fell soundless onto the floor. Only then, she glanced my way. She glided towards the door, brushed my lips with a kiss, and gently tugged on my hand.

'Come on, what took you?'

I was led into the room. Gwen extinguished the light, and for the first time I entered the cage of her embrace. My life had changed irrevocably, and that night I would not have swapped places with anyone. After, she watched as I jerked twitching from side to side, beneath her, inside her. Like a fish thrashing on the river bank, gulping in painful, suffocating air.

At work the next day, I still had her taste in my mouth. I could smell her on my skin, remember her every move. Sleeping alone would prove impossible. I let my nursing duties suffer for the first time, feeling incredibly distracted. When I went to the hospital chapel, playing my eyes over the coloured tiles, I was now imagining how I would go home and make love to Gwen.

CHAPTER SEVEN

One week passed at M'tarfa, and then another. Anna McHardy had departed for Egypt in a blaze of kisses, tears, and bear hugs, but still there was no sign of Nan. I was finding it hard to sleep, my mind unable to relax. Too many thoughts jostled noisily for attention, mostly of Nan, but also of work. It was hot in the barracks, and an echo chamber; every sound from above reverberated inside my room. There were also the mosquitoes. One particularly stubborn character pestered me for hours before landing, teasing, on the sheet above my crotch. I was faced with an awkward decision, to punch or leave it alone. I settled for the punch, and watched in resentful agony when it buzzed malignantly away.

The initial admissions to F Block comprised mainly of diarrhoeas and dysenteries, as expected. That cold shudder and sweat of the patient quickly became familiar, and we also saw cases of Sand Fly, Scarlet, and Undulant Fever. Anna had briefed me well, with ward management and duties easily controlled. I put in longer hours than expected; it provided a welcome distraction, and Matron seemed pleased with my efforts. She told me how Sister McHardy had said I'd be a safe pair of hands. With the notes that Anna had left, I was able to confirm diagnosis and treatment with relative ease.

It was after completion of an 8 p.m. shift, and finishing all the paperwork, that I headed wearily out of F Block. A figure leaned against a column of St. Oswald's Chapel, within the hospital grounds, half turned away from me. A loose khaki shirt blew in the wind and there was something in the posture that I recognised immediately. The head was lowered, but I knew I wasn't mistaken. All my tiredness disappeared in an instant.

'Nan!'

I ran, stumbling, to hold her in my arms, attempting to kiss, talk, and smile, all at the same time. 'You made it!'

'Hello Harry!' Our lips joined, a meeting of tongues. 'It took forever, didn't it! They wouldn't tell me when I'd be transferred until this morning, so I couldn't let you know. But I'm here now!'

I buried my face into her hair, greedily breathing her in.

'You look, smell, and feel, fantastic. I've missed you so much.'

'And how are you, Harry?' She smiled. 'How have you been?'

'Fine. Fine. But I'm better now.'

'That's good.' Nan held me away from her, studying my face, while I stood grinning like an idiot. 'And now I can start to show you the island.'

'I've been looking forward to it.'

She lent into me. The memory of her lips, that mouth, had not done Nan justice. I bent down and kissed the smooth nape of her neck.

'Come on Nan, let's go to my room.'

'Isn't that a bit risky?'

'Probably, but I don't care, I've missed you so much! It's at the end of a block, so we should be able to slip in undetected. It'll be dark soon.'

I placed my arm around her shoulders, her own about my waist. We walked out of the hospital gardens and slowly began the climb up St. David's Road. There was not a soul around, as if fate itself conspired in our favour. Deep orange light faded quickly from the day. When I looked at Nan, I felt invincible. Nothing could or would go wrong.

'So how's it been in Valletta?'

'Much the same, really. Work's been fine and I haven't been out often since you left. But I did see Dicky once - he said to say "hello".'

'How's he?'

'Much the same, as well. Which ward did they give you here? I wasn't sure where to find you.'

'F Block. Infectious diseases.'

We reached the barracks. The street remained deserted, reassuringly silent.

'Come on, Nan! This is our chance.'

I grabbed her hand and we crept noiseless into the building, into my room. The cabinet was shoved against the door, to prevent anyone from entering, and I was suddenly glad of the tiny window. It afforded us some privacy.

Nan was smiling now, and it was with fingers beating with love that our embrace began. I brushed her hair, copying the way she did it, and stroked my hands along her sides, lightly following the curves of her body.

'You,' she sighed.

Every sensation felt different with Nan. Everything felt better.

'You don't know how much I've missed you.'

'I think I do, Harry.' She kissed me on the lips. 'I'm really glad to be here.'

She spoke quietly and carefully began to unfasten the buttons on my shirt, one at a time, pausing to kiss both nipples. I stiffened at the flick of her tongue. My bare arms were released, gently, before Nan fell to her knees. She unbuckled my belt, I stepped from the trousers, and Nan rested her head against me. My shorts were slowly pulled down, and she brushed the palms of her hands over my buttocks.

'I've been waiting to do this,' she whispered.

Naked, I lay on the bed. Her gaze never faltered, her smile constant, when she stepped from her own clothes and onto me. We kissed again, tender now, and Nan adjusted her body. Her lips touched my neck, my shoulders, my chest, with exquisite lightness, before resting delicately onto my stomach. Excited with anticipation, she then surprised me by listening to the churning of my insides. Nan burst into sudden laughter.

'It's really noisy down here! You should hear it.'

She lay still. A wonderful calm spread around us, filling the little room, and already I could not imagine a life without her.

Later, she drifted asleep pressed against me. My stomach continued to churn. I felt a pain in my leg from where she lay, and it was the sweetest pleasure I had known.

Our free day coincided on the Wednesday of that week, and Nan had already decided where she was going to take me.

'It's got to be Buskett Gardens, Harry. It's not too far away, and it's the only wood on the island. It will remind you of home, of England.'

'That's the last thing I want! I'm happy here on Malta, Nan. With you.'

'Well you're going anyway,' she smiled. 'But I'm glad to hear it.'

We walked briskly through the narrow, winding streets of nearby Rabat, before heading down into the valley. Towering prickly pears lined the roadside, along with purple and red hibiscus, a field of giant sunflowers. Lizards bathed decadently in the sunshine, and I watched as Nan jogged ahead. Her dress was the deepest shade of blue, decorated with a shiver of yellow and white flowers. The fit was tight, showing off her figure, and she looked stunning. I was able to gaze at the backs of her shapely, tanned, legs.

'Come on, Harry,' she sang out the words. 'We'll take all day at this pace!'

We'd set out early in the morning, to avoid the strongest heat. Small birds and cicadas competed with each other to make the most noise, and Nan led me across flower-covered fields, past ornate churches with twin towers that were characteristic of the island, and into a valley filled with miniature pink flowers. The smell was wonderful, and I asked her what it was.

'Thyme, Harry. Wild thyme. They use it to make honey, but the best type comes from Gozo.'

'Where?'

'Gozo. It's a small island north of Malta. The honey's excellent and you'd love the wine. It's got deeper soil, good for the vines.'

'You'll take me there?'

'Of course I will!' She laughed.

'Really, Nan?' I was serious. It seemed somehow of great importance.

'I hope so. It's quiet there, very beautiful. I've only been the once, but I loved it.'

The path began to climb. The terraced fields that we passed now stood empty, and Nan said that this was due to the war. An occasional scarlet butterfly fluttered through the warming air. Green woodland appeared in the distance, at the top of the valley.

'Blimey Nan.' I pointed in amazement. 'It's Dover Castle!'

Poking its head above the trees, a white building shone radiant with warm washes of sunlight.

'That's the Verdala Palace, Harry. We're nearly there, the gardens are just behind it. Come on, I'll race you!'

She broke into a run, and I was happy to follow. When we reached the gates of the palace, I caught up with her. I grabbed Nan close and we kissed for a long time; I'd made a vow with myself, when waiting at M'tarfa, that I'd never pass on such an opportunity. I breathed the smell of her deep inside me.

'Look at the view, Harry,' she twisted around. 'It's my favourite on the island.'

We stood on a rise overlooking the gardens. Silvery pines, olives, and almond trees sloped away from us, the cobalt sea sparkling in the distance. I felt the wind ruffle my hair and Nan pulled me forwards, to smooth it back down. She kissed the tip of my nose.

'So do you like it then, Harry?'

'I love it.'

We turned left, strolling along a narrow dusty path that carried us though shady groves, under the arches of cypress trees, allowing time to admire the explosion of colour from the many plants that flourished here. It was quiet, a cathedral hush after the bustle of Valletta and even M'tarfa, the air now thick with white butterflies. Stately Jerusalem pines watched over us like elders. Carob trees and orange groves provided shelter from the sun. A large bumblebee hovered about my head before disappearing into the shadows.

'See that Nan?' I pointed after it. 'My mother used to say

that means we'll be getting a visitor from abroad.'

'So long as it's not the Germans!' she shot back.

In a corner site, well screened from the rest of the gardens, I spotted a huge old twisted vine that was as thick as an elephant's trunk. It bore not only grapes, but also figs and prickly pears.

'Look at this, Nan!'

The trio of plants had become entangled over the years, and grew as if from one root.

'Could be worth remembering. Well done, Harry. I'm hot now, do you fancy a swim?'

'I'd love one. But I haven't got my costume.'

'Neither have I.'

'Well you'd better show me the way.'

We walked out of Buskett Gardens and back onto the twisting road. A hundred metres of rugged, barren land, past another church, and it delivered us onto the cliffs at Dingli. This time it was me who raced ahead until I reached a sudden drop, staring awe-struck at the horizon. The sea here was a colour I had only ever dreamed of; mostly silver, the faintest trace of blue, and mixed with a pale splash of green. Lost out on its own, a tiny islet flickered in the distance.

'Where's that, Nan?' I waited for her to reach me.

'Fifla. It's nothing really. I've heard your soldiers use it for target practice.'

'The bastards! So how do we get down?'

'Ha ha,' she winked, playful, 'that's one of my secrets. There's a cove near here that nobody seems to know about. It's always deserted.' She took my hand and began walking towards an apparent dead end. An isolated, spartan basilica emerged from out of the solid rock. 'That's the Magdalena Chapel, Harry. I love that name, Magdalena.' The word wallowed and luxuriated on her lips.

I was delighted to spot the pathway that appeared abruptly within the cliff face, only becoming evident once we stood right alongside it. Nan immediately began the long climb down.

'Been coming here for awhile now, always on my own.' She skipped nimbly from rock to rock. 'It's so good to have you with me.'

I struggled after her, slipping and skidding, the water below humming, hissing, surging, whispering, growing ever louder, as we continued our descent. A twist in direction, and suddenly we were arrived at Nan's cove. It was tiny, a miniscule rocky beach hidden by a cleft within the cliff. Nan flung off her clothes, and raced straight into the sea.

When she disappeared beneath the waves, I was struck by a sudden idiotic worry that the water, attracted by her beauty, would claim her for its own. I shivered, the hairs on my arms and neck bristling upwards, breathing stalled, and it was a tremendous relief to watch her resurface.

She walked towards me. I crouched in the shallows, gasping with the shock of cold, and then she was on top of me. Coolness was replaced with familiar heat, Nan's arms reaching behind my head, resting on my shoulders. We spun around in the water. As Nan grew close she brought her hands in, holding onto the back of my head. The salt taste of her skin, the touch of her lips; it was the first time in life that I had experienced complete happiness.

Our next trip was into Mdina, as suggested by Anna McHardy. I could easily have done this on my own, but I'd waited for Nan to arrive. The town was clearly visible from both the hospital and barracks, a compact cathedral splendour against the untidy sprawl of Rabat. It was an imposing sight, surrounded by colossal grey stone walls, the twin towers of the cathedral clearly visible at the highest point.

We walked down a steep dirt track leading out of M'tarfa, careful to avoid the banks of iris-blue flowers and prickly pears. A heavy smell of vanilla clung low to the ground. We passed the usual selection of hibiscus, oleander, and almond trees.

'I like walking, Harry. I like holding your hand.' Nan was in a particularly good mood. Her work had been far less stressful since the transfer to M'tarfa and, of course, we were back together. 'I want to be doing this when we're old.'

'Me too. And I want to be wearing my shorts, flashing my knobbly knees!'

Nan leaned against me, and soon we were climbing the far side of the valley. It wasn't a long walk. Jasmine and tall, skinny palm trees lined the track, which was bordered with terraced fields and more of the tiny pink flowers. There were darting birds and butterflies, and then welcome sandstone shade as we neared the city. The guesthouse Point de Vue was on the right, now a Sergeants' mess, and we chose to enter Mdina through the gate found nearest to this. Nan stopped to pat two statues of growling, fierce-looking lions.

Inside the fortified walls, we were greeted with magnificent architecture that basked in generous splashes of white light. Nan was excited, animated, pointing out various palaces that dotted the narrow streets.

'This used to be our capital Harry, before Valletta was built. The poor people lived outside, in Rabat,' she explained.

The sand coloured walls and closed shutters, the empty streets; Mdina possessed an eerie silence. I could understand why Anna had liked it so much, but a city without noise felt wrong, it made me uneasy.

'There's the Palazzo Saint Sophia. It's the oldest building here. But you must see this.' Nan jogged across the road to a tiny chapel. It didn't look anything special. 'This is the church of St. Roque. It's an important one for F Block, Harry, because he's the patron saint of diseases. You two ought to make friends.'

She lowered her head, making the sign of the cross. 'Now I have introduced you. He will look after you.'

She suddenly noticed that I had remained silent since entering the town. 'What's wrong, don't you like it here?'

'It feels strange Nan, too quiet.'

She frowned, crossing her arms.

'But surely that's a good thing? What could be wrong with that?'

'You're probably right, it's just that I'm not used to it.'

'But after all the attacks, this is wonderful.'

'Well, you've seen more of the action than me.'

The island was fortunately enjoying a continued period of respite. Since the night of my arrival, attacks had been nowhere near as frequent. Nan frowned and walked ahead.

The street opened out into an irregular plaza, Bastion Square. I had soured her good mood, to my regret, and vowed to make an effort to be more cheerful. We continued forward to the edge of the square before climbing steep steps onto the ramparts, allowing us to gaze out over the battlements. It was suddenly easy for me to stop feeling so miserable.

The view was spectacular, providing a similar panorama of the island to that from above the operating theatre. What made it even better was that from here it was possible to see

M'tarfa hospital clearly, a grand sight in my eyes.

'Thanks Nan,' I reached for her hand, kissing the side of her face. 'You're right. This is something special.'

I chose to ignore the gunpost that lurked ominously in the corner of the square.

I only ventured into Valletta when Nan was busy on the wards. She was glad to leave the capital behind, preferring the quiet spots found near M'tarfa. I still enjoyed the atmosphere, but definitely preferred my time spent with her. Dicky had been right about catching something nasty in the Gut, for venereal diseases were becoming increasingly prevalent. I knew this for a fact, because I often ended up treating an assortment of such cases.

The supervision of F Block was a definite success. It seemed that all my previous training had been leading up to this moment, and I was more than ready for it. The Maltese nurses were good, as Anna had predicted, and half the time I didn't need to give them any instruction. Matron was pleased with my efforts and had begun to call me Harold. Just once, I noticed her smile.

I had never known such a run of good luck and didn't take anything for granted. I began to carry Dot's bear again, as a precaution, and he fitted snugly inside my shirt pocket. My father would have laughed at me but I didn't care; I didn't want anything to change, or to go wrong.

Two months had passed since Nan's arrival in M'tarfa and relations between us remained wonderful, deepening, thickening, each day. Our favourite destination became Buskett Gardens, and Nan always carried a bamboo mat, rolled up tightly, for us to lie upon. The other men never bothered to walk this far, preferring to remain in the vicinity of the barracks. The furthest they seemed to venture on foot was the Point de Vue, near Mdina gate, and of course rides were always available for the journey into Valletta. It seemed Buskett Gardens belonged only to Nan and me.

I felt an urgent need to touch her as much as possible, skin sliding on skin, be it holding hands or even our legs entwined beneath a café table. I wanted to somehow melt into her, to become one, and I wanted us to share everything. In the gardens, this seemed possible.

A routine quickly developed. I would always pinch a couple of grapes from a field along the way, and Nan would tell me off. At the gates to the Verdala Palace we kissed, as we did in Valletta whenever approaching our lighthouse. The first thing on arrival was invariably to make love, footsteps quickening in anticipation when we neared our destination. We lay in the hidden corner next to the twisted vine, its fruit just an arm's length away.

Two months had passed, and I couldn't put it off any longer. I had to say something, but wasn't sure how to begin. Nan sat hugging her knees, smiling.

'We have no secrets Harry, that's important,' she said. A white butterfly cut through the air, lurching between us. 'I know I can tell you anything.'

I stretched to wipe a bead of sweat from her naked breasts, flattening the tiny hairs on her skin, then pressing the finger to my lips.

'There's one thing I have to tell you, Nan. It's been troubling me all the time, and I didn't know how to say it.'

'What is it?' She turned to face me, suddenly anxious. I struggled to find the right words, to continue with my admission.

'I was seeing someone back in England. But it's over. It's

been finished for some time, and that's why I wanted to get away.'

She remained silent. Nan sucked in her bottom lip, twirling hair around her fingers.

'Really Nan, it's finished. It means nothing.' I placed my hand on the small of her back, but she flinched away. The hand flopped useless onto the mat. 'Nan, you mean everything to me. Everything.'

A salt tear appeared at the corner of her eye, spilling over and down her face. She looked straight ahead, at the ground, the canopy of leaves, anything but me.

'Harry, why didn't you tell me?'

'I was going to. I…'

'Did you live together?' Her voice was altered, sharpened. 'Yes. But...'

'For how long?'

She was crying freely now. I tried to touch her, to hold her, but Nan sprang to her feet. Out of reach. She wiped her tears with forced, jerking movements, at the same time grabbing for her clothes.

'How long?'

'I'm not sure. A couple of years. But it is over, I'm telling you the truth. I wouldn't lie to you, Nan.'

'Just not tell me, is that right Harry?' She was nearly dressed. Her skirt was pulled up quickly. 'I can't do this, Harry. I trusted you. I thought we had something special, something pure. It's ruined.'

'It's not, Nan. It's still there,' I protested. 'I would have finished things in London, but I was going away. I didn't expect to meet anyone. God, I didn't know someone like you even existed.'

She froze, one moment, and then grabbed for her shoes.

Nan continued to speak in something approaching her normal voice.

'I am a Roman Catholic, Harry. You know that.' I glanced at the cross around her neck, back to her eyes, pleading. 'You are not. This has been a big problem for me, but I thought we'd get around it somehow.'

'I do believe in God, Nan.'

'It's not the same, Harry. And now this, this revelation. I'm sorry, but I'm not sure I can do this any more. Maybe we shouldn't see each other, I don't know. I'm going now. Goodbye.'

She turned her back and walked away.

'Nan.'

I called out, but she never once turned around. I was left naked, alone, filling inside with a bulging knot of hurt. They call it heartache for a reason; the pain spread from the centre of me, out into the surrounding ribs, and flooding the chest cavity.

CHAPTER EIGHT

My relationship with Gwen was a frantic affair from the outset, never easy. We loved in a hurry, a hint of desperation clinging to our every action, both of us in some way aware that our time together would be finite.

On our first date, we went to see a film in Leicester Square. I have no idea what it was about, because I was far more interested in the hand that explored underneath Gwen's silk blouse. After the lights had turned on, we raced back to her flat and tore each other's clothes off. I had scratches and bite marks for days.

For maybe six months, we couldn't keep our hands off each other. On a weekend, not even food could entice us to leave the lifeboat of her bed, where we remained long into the afternoons. A shared bath would follow, and I always got the tap end. Gwen loved me to sponge every inch of her body, paying particular attention to her calf muscles and feet. I preferred washing her breasts, watching the pink nipples stiffen and rise in response to my touch. I saw less and less of Eric, preferring to spend most of my free time with her.

Training at the National was drawing to a close. I scored top marks in the examinations and this resulted in an introduction to the Matron of St. Peter's London County Council Hospital. It was a real coup, because the LCC hospitals were the best payers of doctors and nurses in the country. Like the National, they had a reputation for excellence.

Matron was friendly and appeared to be impressed with my references. She offered the next available appointment on the spot, a post that would be non-resident, with remuneration commencing at £150 per annum. This would increase to £260 on completion of training. Things were looking up. Finally, I would have some money.

When I wasn't working, I usually managed to stay with Gwen, rather than at the Guilford Street lodgings. The transfer impending, it seemed foolish to pay two rents and we now decided to share a flat. I was consumed with the idea of her; she remained a foreign being, someone that I could never fully understand, but I didn't care a jot. I was in awe of her impulsiveness and apparent independence, determined to show that I would be the one person to stay with her. I would prove myself a man. In truth, my biggest concern was that I should continue to share her bed. The decision to move was also prompted by Gwen's dragon of a landlady, who disapproved of overnight guests. We had become expert at walking up and down the stairs in unison, but she still managed to catch us out. It felt good to be leaving her sharp tongue behind.

Flat hunting was an exciting prospect; at last I felt like a real grown-up, and not someone pretending. It was probably our finest hour, our life together still rife with possibility and the thrill of an adventure. It did not really matter where we should end up in London, the simple fact that it would be our first shared home was enough. Before it all went wrong.

We were lucky, and managed to find accommodation quickly. 36 Elsham Road was in the west part of the city, one chunk of an attractive four-storey terrace. The road ran parallel to Holland Park, near to Shepherds Bush Green and Kensington High Street. Rent was set at a fair seventeen shillings and six pence per week, rates included, plus whatever gas and electricity that we used.

Our flat was located on the ground floor, the front door

leading directly into the sitting room. It was bright inside, the high ceiling decorated with attractive plaster cornices. The wooden chairs and dining table had seen better days, as had the faded brown carpet. Everything looked worn, a little tired out, but I was particularly taken with one aspect of this room; the bay window had white wooden shutters on either side, instead of curtains. This seemed wonderfully extravagant and different, definitely worthy of a woman like Gwen.

We were both surprised that the living room led into the bedroom. Here, in pride of place, a huge wooden bed took up most of the space. I winked at Gwen and she smiled. There was an immense mahogany wardrobe in the corner of the room, a good-sized set of drawers. The dressing table mirror reflected directly onto the mattress.

Kitchen and bathroom were situated to the rear of the flat. Gwen was quick to notice the cast iron bathtub on claw legs, and neither of us cared that the kitchen was tiny. We arranged to move in immediately.

Mr. Porter became our new landlord. A short, stout, gentleman, he lived with his son in the basement flat, in dark rooms crammed full with furniture and souvenirs from time spent living abroad in India. I loved his coloured bedspreads, painted a vivid scarlet and black. He had worked on a tea plantation for many years, before returning to London and investing his savings in property.

Mr. Porter possessed a kind, generous, smile, to accompany an easy-going disposition. He sported a grey toothbrush moustache and was never seen without a red cap that covered his balding pate. There was something in his manner that made you like him immediately. He told us how he had married a lady much younger in years, who provided him with this son before promptly eloping with one of the tenants. He was sixty years old, and proud to possess all of his own teeth. This fact, he attributed to the healing properties of tea.

Moving to Elsham Road, I felt a sudden foolish maturity. It seemed that everything in my life was now in order - I had the job, the woman, and even the future. Everything was in the right place, and I never once stopped to consider if any of this was what I actually wanted.

My time at the National came to an end. I had enjoyed the training and felt sorry to leave, but we had a suitably drunken send-off that Eric Reynolds managed to attend. He even succeeded in pairing off with the beauty in our year, one Margaret McGrath.

The new post at St. Peter's continued to agree with me, and I flourished on a fifty-six hour week. Here, we received a very thorough training in medicine, surgery, dermatology, and venereal diseases, all excellent preparation for the impending onset of war. As trainee nurses, we were often invited to scrub up and assist in the operating theatre, an unusual practice at a time when student doctors performed such tasks. Breakthroughs in treatments were currently being attained through the introduction of new sulphonamide antibiotics, and it was an exciting period to be involved with the health service.

We were also sent to public mortuaries, and to observe autopsies on bodies that had been pulled out of the River Thames. This comprised part of our training in anatomy, but the stink from bloated, rotting, flesh caught in the back of the throat. Gwen complained that it clung to my clothes and hair, insisting that I wash thoroughly before allowed anywhere near her. Our lovemaking grew less frequent.

Based in the East End of London, I now had a new part of the city to explore. During lunch hour or after work, I took to walking on my own, attempting to soak into the city. I considered myself a Londoner now, no longer a boy from Folkestone, and tried to immerse fully into its culture. This was the new me, and I rarely ventured south to visit my parents.

I liked the Whitechapel Road, its elegant wide sweep, and the vast selection of bars. Eric occasionally joined me in the Grave Maurice pub. Commercial Road, Mile End, Stepney; it was all good. The one place I never enjoyed was Cable Street, where the wind carried with it an air of menace. There was something about it that made me tense, and I always tried to avoid it.

A considerable Jewish population lived in the area immediately surrounding the hospital, and I quickly discovered them to be marvellous family people. They took great care of young and old alike, only using St. Peter's when there was really no other alternative. The hospital retained three men to carry out their long established custom of watching over the dead, and an intense competition was evident between these men.

Hospital employees were often approached for information of recent deaths, with gifts offered in exchange. It was a well known practice, ignored by our superiors, and I was sometimes able to bring expensive food and drink home for Gwen. She had a taste for the fine things in life, good wine and French champagne.

It was at this time that Oswald Mosley and his army of thugs began to march through the East End. Taunting and always provocative, he arranged anti-Semitic meetings in the support of Fascism, believing that Hitler would one day rule

England. Several pitched battles were the result, including a particularly nasty one fought on Cable Street. The Jews retaliated after great provocation, assisted by numerous sympathisers, and hospitals in the area were left to pick up the pieces.

Many of those wounded ended up in St. Peter's, and many were seriously drunk. The weapons used included bicycle chains, iron bars, pickaxe handles, and bricks. Some of the injuries sustained were terrible. We resented having to care for the Black Shirts, and always made efforts to treat them the last. It was a timely reminder that war would not necessarily be the worthy attraction I had initially supposed, under the guidance of Overton and Hadley. When I arrived home in the evenings, exhausted and bloody, Gwen listened in shock to news of these battered patients.

Time continued to pass, and the threat of war started to creep into everyday life. I was surprised to realise how life with Gwen had quickly begun to feel like one long routine. I had a role to perform at the hospital, my responsibilities as man of the house, and little else. Lust and initial attraction had failed to develop into anything more substantial, and those long afternoons spent in bed were already a thing of the past.

We spoke of the weather, current news, our shopping needs, occasionally cases at the hospital, but nothing else. When left alone, our thoughts would drift to fill the room, making me aware of the deepening distance between us. We didn't go out much, preferring instead to read or listen to the wireless, quietly withdrawing from each other. We had become a habit together, no more, and in my naivety I accepted this situation. I did not know anything different. I had nothing to compare our relationship with.

One of my colleagues at the hospital, George Ellis, became a member of Mosley's Black Shirts. He made several attempts to convert the rest of us to this cause, with a total lack of success, and it seemed ironic when his position as Territorial Soldier made him one of the first to be called to the colours. It amused us that he'd have to fight against the very beliefs he condoned, and I bought his bicycle at a knocked-down price. I thought he deserved to be fleeced.

I was able to cycle to work, far preferable to a crowded bus or tube ride. The route was a scenic one, encompassing Notting Hill, Marble Arch, Oxford Street, and then onto Whitechapel Road. When traffic was slight on a Sunday, I would pedal furiously all the way, racing against the clock in an attempt to better my quickest time. It was on one such occasion that I first noticed men digging air raid shelters in parks, and erecting surface shelters in the streets. I screeched to a halt, making sure I wasn't mistaken. It was a sobering sight, finally convincing everyone of the nearness and certainty of war. Gwen and I had something new to talk about. We began to grow worried, not least for the safety of her daughter, Diana.

Our fears were confirmed when Hitler attacked Poland and, on 3 September 1939, a declaration of war against Germany was announced. The city felt restless. We all expected terrible things to happen immediately, such as gas attacks, mass air raids, or invasion from the sea. We had visions of Germans marching down our streets, painting swastikas on our churches. Gwen and I decided that it would be sensible for her and Diana to live with my family in Folkestone. As much as anything to do with the war, we needed a break from each other.

They had met just once before, and it had not proved a great success. After the move to Elsham Road, I had considered it a good idea for my family to meet with Gwen, to show off the success I was enjoying in London. She had been less enthusiastic, but eventually allowed me to convince her.

Two hours by train had brought us to Folkestone Central, leaving only a short walk to reach Park Street. Gwen's trepidation now proved infectious. My home town appeared so small and dull after the bright lights of London, I feared that she would think less of me.

Mother had fussed, refusing to sit down, offering endless cups of tea and coffee. Dad sat in the corner, silent, apparently oblivious to our visit. Gwen grew even more nervous, and this manifested itself as she became increasingly outspoken and rude. She talked down to me in front of my parents, repeatedly criticising me, and they believed that I was both manipulated and exploited. Where I had been enamoured by Gwen's city ways, they found her superior air and manners distasteful. Dad frowned at the thought of his own son being bossed around by a woman, and when mother spotted Gwen tipping her undrunk coffee down the sink, that was the final straw. We left soon afterwards.

It was an awful, tense visit, and I was particularly upset not to have gained mother's approval. I placed great value on her opinion. The return journey to London had seemed endless, with Gwen's continued silence far worse than any harsh words. When we jumped off the train at Charing Cross, she muttered, 'I told you, didn't I,' and those were to be her final words of the day. When we returned home to Elsham Road, she locked herself inside the bedroom.

It was a measure of how bad things now appeared, and how poor relations were between us, that she chose to move to Folkestone. The possibility of mass bombing on London, together with the dropping of enemy paratroops, seemed a more immediate concern than invasion from the sea. The prospect of getting away from each other, at least just for a break, appeared too tempting to refuse. We were bored with each other, no more, but the feeling of missing out, being cheated from future happiness, had slowly bled into resentment. We should have broken up there and then, but I was too naïve to realise. Maybe Gwen was just too worried, scared of being left on her own once again.

It was another Sunday morning, while enjoying the cycle ride to work, when I heard my first air raid siren. There was an unusual brightness to the day, a slight nip in the air to sharpen the nerve endings, and I felt wonderfully alive. The wind rushed past my head as I sped along Marble Arch, and then the siren cut into me, beginning its scream. Braking to a halt, I was unsure what to do next.

Police and air raid wardens appeared suddenly, scurrying like little black ants, to shepherd everybody present into the nearby Cumberland Hotel. I was made to leave my bike and hurried along with the flow of people, down steep stairs, into the hotel basement. The door clanged shut behind us.

We were packed tightly together, a smell of fear dirtying the already scarce air, only for nothing to happen. Nothing at all. Nobody spoke and time appeared to stand still, to shiver and freeze with the rest of us. This was terrible for me - I was gripped rigid in the straightjacket of claustrophobia.

I wanted to scream, to pound the walls, to punch noses and force my fellow inmates aside. I needed to escape. Sweat drenched through my clothes and I fought for self-control. I couldn't do a thing. It was awful. The man on my right tried to start a conversation, but I was beyond words. My scowl soon stilled his tongue. A child began to cry and I knew just how he felt.

The eventual all clear rang as the sweetest of sounds. I felt immense gratitude to rush up the stairs and back out into the daylight, to reclaim my fallen bicycle. It lay untouched where I had left it. I actually prayed to God, a short message of thanks, while pedalling onwards to St. Peter's. It was then that I knew the war had finally arrived, with air raid sirens quickly becoming a familiar, dreaded sound.

We soon received confirmation from my mother that it would be all right for Gwen and Diana to board with her, 'under the circumstances'. She had written these words more boldly, an act of defiance, for my understanding only. She'd do this for her son, but she wasn't happy about it.

I felt a measure of surprise to experience complete lack of sorrow at Gwen's imminent departure. It had not been so long ago that we considered ourselves inseparable, and I still remembered this. I didn't know how I could change things, to improve relations between us, and I wasn't sure that I wanted to. Waving Gwen and Diana off from platform two of a crowded Charing Cross Station, I was actually saying goodbye to our short period of contentment.

The Elsham Road flat was reluctantly relinquished. I had enjoyed living there, and felt sorry to leave Old Porter and his quiet son, but it was too big for me alone. A colleague from the hospital, Reg Marriott, had offered cheaper accommodation. I now moved into a room in the big house that he shared with his wife and parents in Hackney.

Training at St. Peter's continued with business as usual. There were many wards and lectures to attend, and I now had nothing to distract from my studies. It was early in 1940 when the final examinations arrived.

Dot's lucky bear sat on the edge of my desk throughout all the written papers. He nestled in my breast pocket during the orals, and he had lost none of his good fortune. I worked hard and passed with ease, successfully enrolled as State Registered Nurse number 501. When I told Gwen this news, she hardly seemed bothered until I told her about the pay rise. I had been offered a new position and remained happily employed at the hospital.

A stalemate was evident on the war front, with nothing much happening in the city. A blackout was enforced at night-time, tattered dusk replacing pale, washed-out days, but it was still possible to venture out in the evenings. I was able to socialise with Eric again, who obviously bore no hard feelings about my previous disappearance. He had been busy himself and carried on dating Margaret McGrath.

We continued to frequent the café of Overton and Hadley, but where Spanish slogans had been painted onto the walls, new posters now appeared. CARELESS TALK COSTS LIVES. WALLS HAVE EARS. The sense of imminent danger contributed a liberating, reckless, atmosphere to the city. We were regularly invited to parties, and I felt excitement at this rediscovered freedom. Our jaunts about the city were better than ever.

Only those with close blood relatives were allowed to visit coastal towns, but I tried to get to Folkestone once a week. Each time, the atmosphere at Park Street grew noticeably worse. Rationing of food, fuel, and clothing, was then upon us, but this did not explain the obvious bad feeling between Gwen and my family. Nothing was spoken of directly, which came as some relief. It was far easier for me to maintain a silence than trigger confrontation or a great argument. I wanted to remain living on my own. I grew to dread these visits, not missing Gwen at all, but experiencing considerable guilt at dropping her onto my mother.

Weeks passed. It was a filthy night, with air as chill as seawater and streets that trembled with rain, when I discovered Gwen huddled shivering on my doorstep. She wore her pale blue blouse under a thin jacket, a fitted black skirt, and stockings; these were clothes that she knew I admired, but far too inadequate for such a night. Her hair was plastered flat to the sides of her head, and mascara had run in two broken lines down her face.

'Hello Harold.' She attempted, and failed, at a smile.

'What are you doing here, Gwen?' My face has always betrayed my true emotions. I was a useless liar, and this was no exception.

'I can see you're pleased to see me.' She stood, great gobs of rain falling from her jacket and onto the ground.

'Of course I am darling,' I lied. 'I'm just surprised. Why are you here?'

'Let me in, first. We need to talk.'

We did not touch. I unlocked the door with a sinking feeling, my hands wanting to shake, and showed her inside. Water continued to run freely from our clothes as she followed me up the stairs.

Inside my room, Gwen sat heavily on the bed. I watched the damp from her clothes spread into the blanket as a slow stain. I hung my own coat onto the back of the door and sat at the desk, twisting around to face her. No words had been spoken since entering the house. Gwen coughed, twice.

'I've got to move back to London, Harold. I can't stand it

any longer. Your mother is driving me mad!'

'How? And what about Diana?'

'She's suffocating me! It's your family and we just don't get on. Diana is fine, though. It's better for her down there.'

I remained silent.

'I can't go on like this any longer, Harold. Say something! Don't you want us to be together?'

'Of course I do, Gwen,' I repeated the lie. 'But I thought we'd discussed all this. It was you who wanted to move.'

'I know. I know.' Her voice grew louder. 'But I've tried, and I can't do it any more! I'm sorry.'

She abruptly burst into tears, an event I invariably struggled to deal with. I crossed the room to hold her, our first contact, and Gwen pressed her head against my chest. My arms felt stiff and useless. The damp from her hair spread a chill deep inside.

'All right, Gwen. We'll sort something out. Are you hungry? Have you eaten? Let's get you out of those wet clothes.'

I handed her my dressing gown, averting my eyes while she undressed quickly.

'Thanks, Harold. That's better. Could you get me some tea and toast?'

I went downstairs to the kitchen, leaving Gwen alone in my room. When I returned up the stairs, she had climbed into bed.

'Here you go, darling.'

She chewed dryly, without speaking. I was working out a plan.

'Well we can't stay here, Gwen. It's not big enough, as you can see, and it would be unfair on Reg. If you're going to stay in London, we'll have to find somewhere else.'

'I've already done that.' She didn't bother to look at me.

'What?'

'I've found us somewhere. I knew that you'd agree. I'll show you in the morning.'

Gwen was back in my life.

Later, when I climbed into bed I placed an arm about her, pulling close so she could feel me pressing against her.

'I'm too tired, Harold.' She edged away. 'Let's get some sleep.'

I didn't bother to argue.

There were many vacant properties as people left the city in vast numbers. We moved quickly into 18 Marchmont Street, near to Russell Square and Whitehall. It was just a couple of blocks away from The National and Guilford Street, my first home in the city, and I tried to convince myself that this had to be a good sign. But on Gwen's return to London, something indefinable between us had died, never to return. Maybe it was more to do with something that had never been present in the first place, and only now I understood this.

CHAPTER NINE

I could not believe that Nan was gone, out of my life. It felt so wrong. Her reaction was exactly the reason why I'd put off telling her about Gwen, but I felt sure that if she let me explain fully and tell her the whole story then she would understand. I knew we were right together for exactly the same reasons that Gwen and I were not. There was no way that I could allow it to end like this.

I resolved to spend every available hour at the hospital, clinging to the hope of meeting her there. It seemed the best course of action to take, and the staff soon grew accustomed to my continued presence. But I could detect the concern in their eyes, and noticed the little kindnesses that they went out of their way to do for me. Only Matron was oblivious that something was wrong, congratulating me on my efforts. 'You're an example to us all, Harold,' she said, with no idea of the true explanation for my apparent diligence. I was working myself into the ground, punishing myself, risking illness through exhaustion.

Diarrhoeas and dysenteries continued to account for the majority of our admissions, with ward disinfection an ongoing battle. There was a real risk of cross-infection unless standards were kept high, and our laundry department was invariably busy. Presenting diseases began to vary as the garrison personnel grew in size, with cases of tuberculosis and malaria now in evidence. I took on the bulk of the work myself, choosing to forget Anna McHardy's advice to delegate. There was still no sign of Nan, and I needed something to plug the open wound inside of me.

I walked past Nan's quarters every day, both to and from

the barracks. She slept maybe one hundred yards from me and, sometimes, I caught sight of a strip of light escaping from within. It was ridiculous – I felt jealous of that light. I wanted to enter the room, and then her, with a desperate need, but she was beyond me now. An ocean of space separated us, and still I had not seen her since that day in Buskett Gardens.

I wanted to twirl her hair around my fingers, breathe my lips all over her body, to feel her weight, her heat, upon me. I wanted to hold her ankle gently in my palm, to run my hand slowly, deliberately, up to her thigh. I wanted to kiss her mouth, her birthmark. I wanted to talk to her.

I ate in the barracks, tasting nothing, and was asleep with exhaustion before my head had sunk into the pillow. The flies did not bother me now, and I woke bitten by mosquitoes that I'd never seen or heard.

Every morning, returning to work, I imagined Nan sleeping in her quarters. The blind was always drawn, and I wanted to slide my body beneath or around it, to curl quietly beside her. I wanted to guard her while she slept, to protect her, to watch over all her dreams.

One dreadful, interminable, week crumbled past, and then another. I had been convinced that through spending my time at the hospital, our paths would have to cross at some point. It was a big place, and unfortunately this had not yet proved to be the case. I was tired, weary of being without her. The hurt had grown worse, fading not at all.

The duty was supposed to be an early finish, 1 p.m., and for once I decided to leave punctually. It was time I returned to Valletta, in the hope of meeting with Dicky. His company was the one tonic that might help to lift my depression, and I was trying to remember the last time we had seen each other. It seemed so long ago.

One of the nurses, Sister Olivia Merciecp, approached my desk. She was a quiet woman, very pretty, and always gave the impression that she was preoccupied with deeper thoughts. She was a good nurse, and I made an effort to smile.

'Sorry to disturb you, Harry. There's someone here to see you.'

'Who is it?' I shuffled the paperwork into three neat piles.

'I'm not sure. A friend of yours, I think. She said it was important.'

She. I leapt from the chair, knocking case notes to the floor, startling the gentle nurse Merciecp.

'Where is she?' I demanded.

'Outside, near the chapel. She said to tell you that she'd wait.'

'Thanks.'

I raced from the ward, oblivious to the turned heads, hoping I wouldn't be wrong. Somebody called out my name, but I wasn't stopping for anyone.

The air felt singed outside, in the gardens. A rose sun sailed high in the sky. The chapel, she'd said, I swivelled quickly, changing direction. To my dismay, there was nobody there. The chapel stood deserted. My hopes, my world, began to fracture at their foundation.

'Hello Harry.'

The voice came from behind me.

'Nan!'

I spun around to face her. She stood maybe twelve inches away, her breath sweet on my face.

'Sorry to disturb you, but I didn't want to miss you. I couldn't leave it any longer.' She paused, looking directly at me, inside me. I saw only her eyes, frozen, unable to move. 'I've been thinking about everything Harry. I can't give you up.'

She fell against me and I held her close.

'I've missed you. So much.' I whispered into her hair, loose strands catching between my teeth.

'You too, Harry. I'm sorry.'

'I should have told you sooner, Nan. But you're back. That's all that matters.'

My arms jumped from her shoulders to the small of her back, holding tightly, then returning to their original position. I didn't want to let go, for fear of losing her again. She stood trembling against me and I kissed the side of her head.

'Fisher!' A sharp voice stung the air, 'You know the rules. We'll have none of that on duty.' Matron stomped past us and into F Block.

'Sorry Nan.' I released her with reluctance, my hand lingering on the curve of her hip. 'I'll be back in a minute. Wait for me here, okay?'

She nodded, smiling. I touched her cheek, quickly, before hurrying back to the ward. Matron stood glaring by my desk, and I crossed the room more slowly this time.

'Sorry, Matron. That won't be happening again.'

She looked at me furiously.

'Well it better not! To think I was coming here to praise you for good work. I could report you, for that!'

She spat the words out, her eyes narrowed and cold. I found myself wondering who had broken her own heart, for surely that could be the only explanation for such anger. She had created a wall about her, impenetrable, deliberately withdrawn from human contact.

'I'm sorry.'

'Just don't let me catch you again.'

I was pleased to notice that someone had picked up all the paperwork, rearranging it tidily onto the desk. It must have been Sister Merciecp, and I made a mental note to thank her. If Matron had seen the mess, I would have been in even more trouble. She made a cursory inspection of the ward and everything appeared to her satisfaction. She was obviously relieved to leave the block, as if embarrassed by my behaviour. I waited a couple of minutes before following her outside.

Nan had walked to the edge of the gardens, standing next to the low stone wall. A tall, old jasmine plant blew white flowers about her feet, and she gazed towards the distant blue of St. Paul's Bay. Cicadas thrummed loudly and she didn't appear to hear my approach.

'Nan.'

She jumped, turning to face me, a smile already on her face. My hand rested briefly on her arm, but I wasn't sure if Matron was still around. Spying.

'Let's get out of here, I'm finished now. Are you off-duty?'

'I'm finished for the day.' She wore her khaki uniform, shirt and trousers, her dark hair tousled by the strengthening wind. 'That's why I came.'

'Well let's go, I don't want Matron to catch us again. Blimey, she can scare you!'

We walked quickly out of the gardens, turning left for St. David's Road. Behind the shade of the wall, I was at last able to hold her, and to kiss her. My hands reached over her body, pulling her against me. I remembered her smell, her touch; nothing felt different between us. Nan remained a perfect fit in my arms.

'I bet Matron's still watching, Harry.' She took hold of my hands. 'All bitter and twisted. She's probably jealous!'

I bent to kiss her again, our hips touching, but she stepped backwards.

'Harry, can we go to Buskett Gardens?'

This time, we walked together. Nan leaned against me, her head resting on my shoulder, my arm curled around her waist. We walked slowly, stopping often for long, exquisite kisses. When I grabbed a handful of grapes, we fed them to each other, dropping the ripe fruit into hot, moist mouths. We did not speak, simply happy to be reunited. Nan and I came together like a force of nature; I knew that this was the only woman for me, the one that I'd been waiting for.

'What are you thinking, Harry?' We neared the Verdala Palace, the pale stone of the building blanketed in a net of shadow.

'That I'm happy.'

'Me too. I couldn't not see you.'

'I'm so glad. I was getting worried. I've missed you so much Nan, I was spending all my time at the hospital, hoping to catch you there. To explain.'

She stopped walking, placing a finger gently over my lips. 'Not now, Harry. We can talk later, another time.'

We reached the gardens, turning in unison along our normal path. A delicious anticipation charged that walk under the trees to our hidden corner, to make things right between us. We hurried to undress and I sat down first, sprawled onto the pile of clothes. Nan didn't carry the bamboo mat. I pulled her onto me with deep, rhythmic strokes. Our lips never parted from each other.

We lay in the shade, skins glued with perspiration. Nan

continued to lie on top of me.

'There's something I've got to tell you, Nan. It's more important than last time.'

'Harry, no. Let it wait, not today.' She appeared worried, studying my face intently. She shifted her body off me and sat upright. Instinctively, her arms wrapped about both knees.

'I can't. I love you.' I had never spoken such words before. I had never wanted to.

'What did you just say?'

'I love you, Nan. I love you!' It was such a relief to breathe life into these words, to release their power. I felt a quickening lightness inside and smiled, an open, honest smile, revealing everything.

Nan lay down beside me, burying her face against my chest.

'What is it, Nan? What's wrong?' I feared at this reaction.

'I love you too, Harry.' She struggled to speak, still hiding her face. 'I wasn't going to tell you yet. It's too dangerous. What if something happens to one of us?'

'It won't Nan. It won't.'

I sat idly stroking her hair. A smell of oranges washed through the air, the wind blew cooler now. A butterfly landed on the vine, fluttering wings like applause, and I believed every word that I spoke.

CHAPTER TEN

I walked to work early the next morning, enjoying the best mood I had felt for a long while. The sun already warmed a sapphire sky, and birdsong sounded louder than usual. A scrawny black cat crossed my path and I wished it a cheerful 'good day'. It was one of those crystal days, the air so clean you could see for miles. I imagined I could hear the gasp of the sea.

Stepping into the hospital gardens, I jumped at the air raid siren. That dreadful, ominous noise had followed me from London and I felt my stomach tighten in recognition. It was the first time I'd heard it for weeks, and I wondered what could be happening. Glancing up to the roof of the hospital, several figures had already begun to collect. I rushed up the stairs to join them.

On top of the operating theatre, all men stood facing the direction of Valletta. Nobody moved. A sound of distant explosions distorted the air about us, sending tremors throughout the building. I heard somebody mutter 'not again', another voice 'it's starting', and I walked forwards, to see what they were talking about.

It wasn't possible to distinguish individual ships and buildings around the Grand Harbour, but we watched in dismay as columns of dirty black smoke rose spiralling from burning dock installations, angry red flames licking the horizon. It was possible to make out the shadows of enemy planes attacking through the flak, the white puffs of anti-aircraft barrage, followed by popping sounds of retaliation. 'Here we go again, lads,' a further voice spoke. We all watched transfixed until the air raid was over. We could not bring ourselves to move away.

I was late into F Block for the first time, where my colleagues were hard at work. Quick inspection revealed that Sister Merciecp obviously had everything under control, and I donned my tunic quickly.

'Sorry Olivia,' I apologised. 'I got caught up watching the action.'

'I guessed that Harry. You'll be surprised how quickly you get used to it.'

The ward round was half complete when the siren began again, heralding another attack. I wanted to watch, but nursing duties had to take precedence. I was supposed to be in charge, not swanning off at every hint of action.

The staff began to place mattresses quickly over any supine patients, and I joined them in this task. Several of the casualties were able to move and Olivia Merciecp shepherded these outside, to the slit trenches. We had rehearsed this procedure many times. Once all the necessary mattresses had been repositioned, to an accompaniment of curses and groans, I realised that each and every one of the nurses had left the building. I was on my own. Claustrophobia ensured that I was going nowhere near a trench.

'All right, Farrell?' A head of curly dark hair nodded weakly. 'It will soon be over.' I patted the side of his bed.

'And you Robinson? How you doing under there?'

'It stinks, this mattress. But I'll live.'

I felt sorry for him, caught under a haze of carbolic acid. 'Good man.'

'Aren't you going outside, sir?'

'No. I'm staying here with you.'

I sat at the desk while the siren continued to scream.

Clouds of white dust twirled in the air, disturbed by further explosions. The ward would need even more tidying, and I cursed the old limestone of F Block. It seemed to require a never-ending clean up. I ran my eyes throughout the room, checking that no beds had been moved accidentally, all patients remained comfortable. I felt for Dot's bear in my pocket.

It was not long before an all clear rang out, the staff and mobile patients returning quickly. By noon the ward had resumed normal function. At this point in time, all our occupied beds were located on the ground floor. The first floor stood empty, awaiting further enemy action.

When Matron walked into the Block on her usual ward inspection, anxiety pinched at her features, her forehead creased with fresh wrinkles.

'So how did it go this morning, Harold? Any problems?'

'No, Matron. We did everything as instructed. The staff were great, but they've done all this before.'

'Yes. That's good.' She appeared distracted, placing one hand on my arm. I jumped - I couldn't help it, I couldn't have been more surprised if the King of England had asked me for dinner. 'It's starting again. I hoped that it wouldn't, Harold.'

'At least we escaped, up here at the hospital.'

'But the casualties are coming already. Surgical is working flat out. They've had one amputation already. The attacks are brutal, Harold.'

I thought about Nan. It was the ward that she worked on.

'Was it like this before, Matron?'

'Yes, but worse. I'm afraid it's all going to start up again. They always go for the harbour first, to cut off our supplies. You wait, the attacks will get frequent now.' She sighed wearily. 'Well if everything's all right, I'd better be on my way.'

I was beginning to understand her hardness. It was partly a survival mechanism, to withstand the traumas of war.

The afternoon passed without incident on F Block, but more news came trickling through concerning the morning's casualties. There had been some terrible injuries, with Surgical operating at capacity. Poor Nan was caught up in the thick of it, and I wished that I could help her.

At night, the siren again sprang into horrible life, and this time I didn't remain inside. I left the barracks quickly, joining the rest of the men who had begun to assemble in a varying state of undress in the courtyard between the buildings. I wore my shorts and shoes, nothing else. It was a hot, sweaty night. I recognised one face from the hospital, standing in darkness on the edge of the group.

'What do you think is happening?' I asked him.

'Same as before mate, just the same.' He sounded bored, suppressing a yawn with one hand and withdrawing a comb from his shirt pocket with the other.

'I wasn't here then. What happened?'

'Right,' he began to tidy his hair, which was layered flat with pomade. 'Well, they'll be trying to sink the boats in the harbour, the ones that actually reached us. And they'll probably be successful - the Maltese dockers always scarper.'

I remembered my driver, the baggage party, on arrival. A loud explosion shook the ground, making me jump, but my companion appeared unmoved. He continued to speak calmly.

'And that'll be the Italians, dropping their bombs anywhere. Probably landed in some poor old farmer's field.'

'Is there anything to see?'

'Not now, mate. Just a few tracers. Soon be over.'

He continued to comb his hair and I asked no further questions. Most of the other men remained silent, eager for their beds.

When the all clear sounded and we returned inside, I couldn't sleep at all. I felt restless, a little afraid, considering the awful possibility of something now keeping me from Nan, an injury, or transfer of duty. Nothing could or would go wrong; I repeated the words like a mantra. Nothing would go wrong. I wondered where she was now, how her day had been, and how long these attacks would continue.

Further raids took place in the morning, edging closer to M'tarfa. The relentless clamour of attack seemed magnified inside F Block, producing a constant drumming in my head. The demented rhythm of war. Enemy planes skimmed above us, a chaos of indiscriminate gunshot reverberating within the hospital grounds. The pilots appeared to be trigger-happy, randomly pockmarking the surface of the main building. Anna had been correct again; the Red Cross certainly provided no safe haven. I thought of Nan all the time, no doubt still busy in Surgical.

During one lull in this action, I made it onto the rooftop. I'd been itching to get out, to prevent the onset of claustrophobia, all morning. Half a dozen men stood waiting, enthralled by the awesome spectacle of it all. The siren kicked off again, and enemy attacks quickly recommenced. Planes swarmed noisily in the air, like angry bees. I watched the sky roar and cry with tears of metal and blood. Sparkling explosions hurt my eyes. Black and white plumes rose thickly about the island, particularly from over Valletta, where the horizon smouldered in the distance. It was mesmerising, impossible to drag yourself away. Time lost any real meaning.

'Over there! Ta Qali' someone shouted. We watched four of our Hurricanes destroyed on the ground at the airfield, bursting into flames. A fighter flew low to retaliate, too late, and was forced into attempting an emergency landing. He came in much too fast, the front of the cockpit crumpling on hitting the floor, and another inferno resulted. No ground staff appeared to assist him; he was left to the fire and inevitable death.

More enemy planes joined the attack, climbing and swooping unchallenged. It was happening so close to the hospital and they were in complete control, free of any obvious engagement. The ground winced as each bomb fell, hitting its target with a cruel disheartening accuracy, and soon became scarred with multiple craters.

That night, again I couldn't sleep. The sound of snoring drifted noisily into my room, an occasional fart, while a cat miaowed loudly outside the window. I still hadn't seen Nan. My mind refused to switch off; I kept thinking about the attacks, the casualties, and the hospital. Surgical must have been the hardest of the wards to work. The luminous green hands on my watch turned slowly, and I tossed and turned with increasing frustration. There was no point lying in bed, the air inside the barracks as thick and suffocating as water. I put on some clothes and left the building, deciding to take a walk.

The moon hid above a sky weighed low with smoke. No stars were visible and all lights remained blacked out - I'd travelled a long way to encounter another Blitz. The streets were deserted, a welcome cool, and I twisted between three or four of the barrack blocks to reach the edge of town. Staring into the dark towards a soundless sea, my thoughts were only of Nan.

I wondered whether she was able to rest, to sleep, and if she was thinking of me. I could only guess at how difficult the nursing must had been - so far, duties on F Block had remained much the same. I hoped that she was coping all right.

I thought about our time together, our reconciliation. It seemed bigger than the war, more important, and I silently repeated the words 'nothing could go wrong.' Our love was indestructible. It had to be. It was the only thing in my life that made any sense.

'Hello, Harry.' A voice sounded in the blackness.

'Nan?'

A shadow approached from a nearby doorway.

'I thought I'd find you here. I couldn't sleep.'

'Neither could I. Blimey, Nan! I was just thinking about you.'

'And I was thinking of you.'

We came together as relaxed, as natural, as an old couple. She reached for both my hands.

'I'm so pleased to see you, Harry. It's been tough on the ward.'

'I bet! I've been wondering how you were doing.'

'I don't really want to talk about it. Just hold me, will you?'

I placed my arms around her and pulled her to me. Our bodies touched all over, but there was nothing sexual in this act. I buried my face into Nan's hair; she pressed her head against my shoulder. Calmness spread between and around us, a feeling of security and peace. No further words were spoken. When I walked Nan to her door, we kissed with unforgettable tenderness.

Admissions started early in the morning on F Block, increasing dramatically over the following days. All men suffered identical symptoms; headache, sore throat, a raging fever, and stomach cramps. These quickly developed into chills, sweating, the rankest of green diarrhoeas, and even delirious muttering. Carpet bombing of the airfield had damaged the underground sewers. This had led to contamination of our water supply, and we now had an outbreak of typhoid on our hands.

All energies were directed at keeping the patients comfortable, attempting to prevent the temperature rise that brought about a crisis in the disease. After this, the patients would either recover or die. I had no prior experience of the nursing.

Ward disinfection became even more paramount than usual, to avoid the spread of typhoid. I was glad that the screening of our windows and doors remained in good shape, to prevent flies from contacting any excreta and causing a further spread of disease. The staff worked terribly hard, cleaning, providing cool sponge baths, and making sure that all patients remained adequately hydrated. We needed the beds on the first floor, and I was worried to diagnose tuberculosis in one of the patients. Cases of cerebrospinal meningitis also began to present, which I had treated at the National in London.

This always seemed to follow a septicaemia, an infection of the blood, and symptoms were unmistakable; headache, nausea, vomiting, together with stiff neck, chills, and fever. These patients were invariably irritable, confused, and one of them suffered from violent convulsions. I had to protect him from self-injury during a particularly nasty fit; he scratched my face to pieces, it was bloody hard work.

Lumbar puncture was necessary for the diagnosis and correct treatment of meningitis. This procedure now became my responsibility, and Matron provided hollow needles that were appropriate for the task. The other nurses worried how these were awfully big in size, and only Sister Olivia Merciecp had sufficient confidence to volunteer assistance.

The patient was made to lie in a foetal position, and I counted carefully to the space between the third and fourth lumbar vertebrae. I always did this out loud, with Olivia double-checking, for a mistake would have unthinkable consequences if I damaged the spinal column. The skin of the lower back was swabbed meticulously with alcohol and stretched tight. I then had to be extremely careful how I inserted the needle, advancing steadily through the dura mater, to avoid hitting the spinal cord.

Cerebrospinal fluid was aspirated from this space. Olivia assisted the patient in physically keeping their knees and head flexed as much as possible, to ensure they did not move. The fluid was sent to the hospital laboratory and results were quick to come back. Treatment could then be tailored precisely to the patient, increasing the prognosis of success. It was a barbaric job that I hated, but there was no one else to do it. I wanted to spend time with Nan, but this was no longer possible.

The attacks on the island continued. Point de Vue was hit, by the gateway to Mdina, with several men from the barracks killed. We had to ignore all this and continue with our work. It was good to be kept well occupied.

I remained in the hospital most hours of the day, returning to quarters only when dismissed by Matron. I slept without moving, exhausted, my bed undisturbed in the morning. At the first hint of daylight, I returned to F Block where work continued in my absence. All of the staff proved conscientious in their efforts. Our patients appeared reasonably comfortable, stable in their disease, and so far we had avoided fatalities. Attacks resumed without fail after dawn, but already this had become normal. As Olivia Merciecp had suggested, it was nothing to get excited about.

There was a lessening in the action during the afternoon. After checking that I wouldn't be missed for a few minutes, I set out in search of Nan. Days had passed since our last meeting, and I desperately wanted to be with her.

It was another scorcher, the ground baked hard beneath my feet. Even the lizards appeared sluggish, slow to get out of the way, when I trudged across the gardens. A scent of jasmine blew across me and I stopped to look at the sea. I liked to watch it every day, noting the changes in colour, and today it was glorious pale silver.

A buzzing vibrated in the air. This was unmistakeably a plane, but it sounded different from usual. The noise grew suddenly louder, transforming into a roar, and then I heard the rat-a-tat of gunshot. An enemy plane sped low over the ground, from the direction of Mdina, and it was heading straight towards me. It took just seconds. I could make out the young face of the pilot, mouth open, his features contorted into a grimace. A string of bullets hit the earth near to where I stood, and only then I started to run.

I sprinted for the shelter of the hospital. More bullets hit the ground, maybe two feet either side of me, and I expected to go down at any moment. The noise was deafening, bludgeoning my ears, and I turned my head to the floor, willing my legs to move faster. Survival was the only thing on my mind. And then suddenly it was over, as quickly as it had begun. Silence returned to the gardens.

I found that I was shaking and couldn't stop. I had escaped injury, unharmed, and deep joy filled into my body. I looked down to discover that I actually stood upon the red cross, and it took a moment to register that someone was calling out. 'Okay, I'm okay.'

A man came stumbling towards me, half falling, like a broken doll. His face was white, one scarlet hand returning to the identical place on his scalp. 'Okay, I'm okay,' he continued to repeat the words. I could not move.

The man reached the cross and fell against me. A strong smell of sweat was mixed with something else. Excrement. And only then I realised that the top of his head was peeled back, like the lid of a tin of sardines.

'You'll be okay, mate, that's right.'

I struggled to hold onto him, afraid of contaminating his wound. There would be a high risk of tetanus infection if it should contact the ground. I managed to lower him carefully, cradling his head in my lap. The blood was beginning to clot, as thick and warm as homemade jam.

'How's that, then? More comfortable?'

He had stopped speaking, and before any help had chance to arrive he was lost. I remained on the ground, staring at his calm, unburdened, face. He looked so young and relaxed, almost happy. I was consumed by the pointless waste of it all, by the thought that it could just as easily have been me.

In the evening, I was finally reunited with Nan. It had been tough returning to the ward, somehow futile, after watching chance killing a man at random. Nan had been told about the incident, and realised that it involved me. She had sent a message to F Block and now we walked from M'tarfa.

'It must have been awful, Harry. I know.' She held onto

my arm with both hands while we followed the dirt track into the floor of the valley. The air was still and heavy, as comfortable as a warm bath.

'It was more real this time, Nan. Too real.' I still wondered why this incident had shaken me so much, for death had quickly lost any strangeness since the voyage from Gibraltar. Like so many other things, we'd just had to get used to it. To accept it.

'I know. Sometimes it just gets to you. I try to turn off, to concentrate only on the nursing duty, but it can be so upsetting. We wouldn't be human otherwise.' She squeezed my arm.

'It just doesn't make much sense right now.'

'It won't.' Nan paused. 'It can't. And I'm glad about that. I wouldn't want to understand it.'

We began to climb the far side of the valley, heading towards Mdina, accompanied by the constant rasping serenade of the cicadas. It would take more than a war to silence them, and I felt so glad to have Nan with me.

'You must have seen some sights?' I asked. 'At the beginning?'

'I did, Harry. Horrible things.'

'Like what?' I needed to know.

'I've tried to forget. There's just one thing that keeps coming back to me, when a building collapsed in Valletta. We were sent to help, into the ruins.' Nan spoke slowly, hesitant. She reached for my hand, our fingers knotting together. 'And it was me who found them. A whole family. The grandparents, parents, young children. I couldn't tell which body belonged to which. I've no idea how many of them there were.'

'I'm sorry.' I held Nan against me, pressing my face into

her hair. She was trembling. 'Are you all right?'

She shook her head, refusing to look at me. I felt her tears soaking into my shirt, on my chest, above my heart.

'What is it Nan?' Gently holding her from me, she had her eyes shut tightly. I kissed both eyelids, catching the tears with my lips, and felt her body begin to relax. 'We're still here, aren't we? That's what matters.'

'I know.' She breathed the words. 'That's why I'm crying.'

We entered the city, my arm about her shoulders, walking slowly along the dark, narrow streets. A gentle murmur of voices was audible behind some of the closed windows and doors, a reassuring sound of everyday life. A smell of cooking, of freshly baked bread, wafted through the air.

In Bastion Square, I kissed her. We stood in silence, hand in hand, leaning against the cool stone of the ramparts. The dark shadow of the hospital appeared quiet behind us, illuminated by a single star, yet bombs continued to fall on Valletta. We gazed at the distant pyrotechnics, the reds and the greens in the sky, but on this night the cacophony of death failed to reach us. There was not a soul around. We stood until the colours grew still.

'I suppose we'd better get back, Nan. In case we're missed.'

'Harry, let's take our time.'

Avoiding the main street, we began to head for home by criss-crossing all of the tiny alleyways, like a small boat tacking the wind. We heard somebody learning the trumpet, obviously a beginner, and in every false note there was a quality of defiance that was somehow triumphant.

In one of the smaller squares, a man and woman were singing folk songs from inside one of the houses. Nan tugged on my arm to stop walking.

'We sang these as a child. I haven't heard them in years,' she whispered, her mouth stretched close to my ear.

The sweet voices rose and fell together, and I imagined Nan as a girl. A pretty, happy, child, filled with life and laughter. I pictured her transformation, year by year, into the beautiful woman standing by my side. I was an incredibly fortunate man. To my surprise, my own eyes now filled rapidly with tears and I needed to blink quickly, to remove all evidence. We stood and listened as the voices fell silent.

'Don't leave me tonight Harry. I want to be with you.'

'I didn't want to be alone.'

It was always a risk to smuggle Nan into the barracks, but on this night it seemed more important than anything. We made it undetected once again, barricading ourselves into the room. I was able to hold her through the night, stroking her back, retracing the words of my love.

Matron arrived early in the morning, with news that the Royal Opera House on Kingsway had been destroyed. A direct hit, the building had caught on fire while its columns collapsed into ruins. A soldier who had been admitted in the night told of watching the backdrops and costumes blazing away. As one of the finest buildings on the island, its destruction angered everybody.

On F Block, we now had sixty patients with typhoid, each of them requiring a high degree of care. The staff continued to work hard, above and beyond the call of reasonable duty, and we had only lost one patient. He was the one who'd also contracted tuberculosis. Matron began to visit us several times a day, obviously pleased with our efforts. She returned to calling me Harold, my previous indiscretion forgiven.

The air raids continued unabated, with disconcerting lack

of a fight back. I watched more Hurricanes destroyed on the ground at Ta'Qali, and the hospital remained a target. I still ventured onto the roof when duties allowed, and once had to take shelter on a first floor balcony. An aerial battle progressed directly above our heads, and several of us watched this rare sight of engagement. The man next to me said that it was far better than any Hollywood film.

The planes chased each other, a game of cat and mouse, covering a large expanse of sky. I thought that our plane was on top, winning, but you couldn't be too sure. It could all change in one second. I watched in delight when a string of bullets tore into the German fuselage, just behind the cockpit.

The battle appeared to be moving east, towards Mdina, but we continued to remain stationary. It did not pay to take unnecessary chances. It was a small piece of shrapnel that spiralled beneath the balcony, entering my companion's skull with a sickening crunch. He fell to the floor at my feet, death inching ever closer. It was another random killing. I had to stay alive; there was so much love to live for. I had to keep on breathing. For Nan.

I was never a shelter man, although few people realised that this was actually due to claustrophobia rather than any great bravery. I saw no reason to explain myself. When the sirens sounded, I always remained on the ward. Those patients unable to move appreciated this presence, that not everyone deserted them to fate. I strolled amongst the beds, chatting above the sometimes thunderous noise of battle, trying to keep the men as calm and relaxed as possible.

In the same week that the Opera House was destroyed, I was patrolling inside F Block while the onslaught continued for longer than usual. All hell appeared to have broken loose, explosions and tremors shaking the building with gloomy regularity. The clatter of gunshot sounded ominously close and then there was a different noise, a wail, becoming shockingly loud. I stopped moving when an inhuman roar pained my ears. I saw windows shaken loose from their frames, beds jolted into movement, and then nothing. A period of blackness followed.

I found myself lying on the floor and trying to breathe. The air was choking with smothering white dust. I didn't know where I was and could hear nothing. My head felt stuffed with giant dressings of cotton wool.

I staggered to my feet when the cloud began to disperse. A door had fallen open and then completely off its hinges. The dust began to settle, revealing the decrepit state of the ward; it was as if the building had burst outwards, with half the windows now missing. A jumble of beds had been shaken to the centre of the room, all occupants either motionless or gesticulating in complaint.

I raced about the ward, checking for injuries. One man's face had become a riot of red, a deep gash in his forehead that would require several stitches, but otherwise he was in one piece. I turned to watch Matron burst into the room through the space where the door had previously stood. Her glasses had fallen off, her hair wildly dishevelled.

'Harold! Thank God!'

My hearing was still affected and I could barely catch her words.

'What happened, Matron?'

'Just tell me, are you all right? Any casualties on the ward?'

'A few cuts and bruises, otherwise we seem to be okay. What was that?'

The battle was still in progress. I began to hear a muffled

siren. Another explosion.

'A bomb, Harold! It hit the roof and bounced off, landing between F and G blocks. Thank God you're okay. I can't quite believe it.'

I looked down in surprise; Matron was holding onto my arm. I struggled to speak, but my mouth was uncomfortably dry.

'A close call. I suppose we'd better start tidying up then.'

It wasn't until evening that the shock began to wear off. I realised I should have been dead - the bomb had hit our roof! I dropped to my knees, resting my head on the thin barracks mattress, and I prayed. For some reason, either fate or pure chance, I had survived again and was extremely thankful for this. Since London, I had stopped living the life of a single man, without concern for my safety. I now had a reason to live, and that reason was of course called Nan. I prayed for the survival of our love.

News from Valletta went from bad to worse. It was taking a hammering, and the Regent Cinema was next to be destroyed. There were over forty reported dead, and a large number of serious casualties including amputations. Death and destruction now came unheralded to the island, and I feared for Dicky's safety. The Regent had been one of his favourite haunts. I managed to take leave of my post for the afternoon, to take a look at the damage for myself, to see if I could find him.

I hitched a lift in the back of an army truck, which dropped me off at the gateway to the city. Immediately, the air felt charred, each breath choking and burning the lungs. Inching slowly along Kingsway, the capital I knew had disappeared.

The Opera House was gone, this was no surprise, but

actually seeing the destruction and ruin was something else. Heaps of rubble appeared in place of buildings and streets, thin columns of dirty grey smoke still rising from out of the wreckage. People clambered over the fallen stone, searching for precious belongings. I recognised the same haunted, weary eyes from the Blitz back in London, and felt glad to be alone. Nan would have been so upset to observe this.

I turned a corner, where young Scouts helped an old lady to cross an obstructed road. A crude sign appeared resting on the rubble, "Business as Usual" and I could see how the storekeeper had fashioned a space in the dirt to sell what was left of his hardware stock. It didn't amount to much more than a few rusty pairs of scissors, but this was unimportant. There was little reason for optimism, but it was good to see his defiance. The people were not beaten yet, despite lack of sleep and serious hunger.

I turned back onto Kingsway, my route blocked. The Regent Cinema had simply disappeared. Vanished. There was no sign of Dicky Fuller when, somehow, I had expected to hear him calling out my name. I couldn't get my head around his absence. I couldn't reach Fountain Street or Fort St. Elmo because the rubble blocking these streets was piled so high. An air raid cut short my visit, and I cadged a lift back up to quarters.

Nan stood waiting outside the barracks when the lorry dropped me off in M'tarfa. She wore her khaki uniform, dark hair tied back for work, and came rushing towards me. She flung herself against me, squeezing the air out of my chest. Her head butted painfully against my chin.

'What is it? What's wrong?' I asked, worried.

'Harry, I thought I'd never see you again!'

'Why? What's happened?'

She pulled back to look at me. Her eyes were wide open, a single tear running down her cheek.

'I can't believe it. It's a miracle. I still can't believe it!'

'Tell me, Nan.'

She grabbed my face, hard, and kissed me on the lips. She pulled my head to her neck, clutching at my shirt.

'You won't believe it, Harry,' she began to explain. 'I went to the church at Mosta, you know, for benediction. The air raid siren went so we stayed inside for shelter. When the attack started, we recited our prayers. It blocked out some of the noise. I was thinking about you, Harry. About us. I was convinced I was going to die, I couldn't stop it. It was horrible.'

'You.' I bent to kiss her but Nan held me away, not wishing to be interrupted.

'That's when it happened! The miracle! A bomb hit us, Harry. It came right through the dome.'

'What?'

'Yes! It seemed to happen so slowly. I saw it come through the dome, and crash onto the floor. It didn't explode, Harry! It didn't explode!'

Nan explained how she had watched in horror while the bomb slithered and zigzagged across the smooth marble floor before finally coming to rest. Nobody had been injured. A soldier had rushed in and out of the building, quickly summoning help, and the bomb was rolled safely outside.

It was indeed a miracle. A second one, if you included the bomb that had bounced off F Block. It was on this day that I began to feel our love could truly be blessed. I dared to believe in Nan's God.

CHAPTER ELEVEN

Convoys could no longer reach the island, and food shortages now kicked in. When even the obnoxious Victory V cigarettes were restricted to five per week, a black market inevitably sprang into life. This traded in every commodity possible that was in short supply. Drinking water became much more limited, and we were each allocated just one quick shower a week. It would have been less of a problem had it remained possible to swim in the sea, but work and enemy action usually prevented such activity.

We still received adequate rations in the Services, but Victory Kitchens were set up for the Maltese population, to economise on food and fuel use. Communal meals were now prepared on a terrific scale, and Nan told me how this had immediately brought about a serious drop in morale among the local population.

From the hospital roof, I watched new Spitfires destroyed on the ground before able to enter into active service, burning fiercely along with our hopes. Enemy attacks continued, undiminished, our ammunition fast running out. Under siege, it simply was not possible to provide much of a fight back.

The siege made nursing conditions difficult. A shortage of water and soap, coupled with lack of food, made it hard to provide adequate care for our patients. With screening on windows and doors now getting damaged, cross-infection was even more of a danger. Large gatherings of staff were no longer permitted, in case of a direct hit depleting the hospital function.

Frequent loss of electricity meant that we sometimes

worked using oil lamps, although this commodity was also in short supply. I was permanently tired, sometimes scared, and yet more fulfilled than at any previous time in life. When on duty or with Nan, the thought of never returning to England brought more comfort than worry.

An average of twenty cases per day were admitted to F Block, with diarrhoeas and dysenteries a constant presence on the ward. We had a steady, controlled, turnover of patients, and I looked forward to inspections from Matron. She had been so nice to me since the bomb hit our roof, and one morning she was accompanied with a visitor.

'Harold, we've someone here to see you. I believe that you've met already.'

Major Merryweather strolled briskly into the room, one hand proffered in greeting.

'Hello, Fisher. Time flies, eh, since you got here? I told you it wouldn't be easy.'

Major Henry Merryweather had followed me from Sliema, the man who had briefed me on arrival. We shook hands and I noticed the tiredness in his eyes. His grip was weak, the palm clammy. He had lost considerable weight.

'Well I'll leave you two alone, then. Other work to be getting on with.' Matron smiled and walked from the building. The Major's eyes followed her out.

'Damn fine woman, that. Worth her weight in gold.'

'Yes sir, I've come to realise. So what brings you here, sir?'

'What?' He appeared distracted, absently scratching the side of his face. 'Yes, I've been transferred myself. We'll be working together now, so you can report directly to me. Well let's have a look at the paperwork then, so I know what's going on.'

He sat behind the desk. I stood behind him and explained about the typhoid outbreak, the cases of meningitis diagnosed.

'Yes, yes. Heard all about it. Heard you did well, too. Well done, Fisher.'

The Major appeared as immaculate as he had on our first meeting. He spoke warmly, never raising his voice, and I was happy to see him again. Some of the superior officers were both arrogant and nasty, but he was never like that. I never saw him lose his cool or speak out of anger.

'How's it been in Sliema, sir?'

'Pretty heavy workload. We've seen a lot of action, being next to Valletta. The psychiatric wards are the ones getting flogged, seems a number of men aren't able to cope with the war. Their wards are packed right out. Most of them are genuine but there's a few trying it on, trying to get themselves sent home. Mind, they must be a little bit mad. There are no boats left to take them, of course.'

We spent the entire morning together, and on this occasion it was my turn to provide the briefing. At exactly 13.00 hours, the Major stood up abruptly.

'That's enough for now, thank you Fisher. I'm impressed. I believe that we shall work well together.'

He shook my hand and marched from the ward, leaving me glowing with this praise. It was always good to feel appreciated.

I met Nan in the evening, our time together now limited to a few snatched hours whenever duties allowed. She stood waiting at the top end of St. David's Road, dressed in the usual khaki. Her face lit up on spotting me and she held her arms out straight, waiting for me to walk into their grasp.

'So how was your day then?' One hand grabbed into hair

on the back of my head, the other pulled me hard against her.

'Can't I just stay like this Nan, and be quiet?'

'No!' She thrust her hips, pushing me away. 'Tell me!'

I explained quickly about the Major.

'Well, you're lucky then. My boss is not so nice.'

'No, Nan. I'm lucky because I have this!' I pulled her tight, squashing her, and she pretended to fight me away, fists punching gently in mock fury. And then we were kissing, always kissing, until a car beeped us from the road.

We walked to Mdina, to escape the oppression of barracks, watching a tangle of red in the sky darken into a sunset of purple and gold. When we stood in Bastion Square, Nan told me how it was just as busy in Surgical, the admitted casualties apparently endless.

'Well, we've just got to live for today, Nan. Nothing else really matters. So long as we've got each other, it can't be so bad.'

'I know, Harry. It helps to talk about it. To be with you.'

'It's the same for me. I just wish we had more time.'

'Impossible, right now. But we will, one day.'

'I hope you're right. You've still got to take me to Gozo.' This island had become an unattainable dream for us, the prospect of visiting a reliable source of hope and wishful thinking.

'I haven't forgotten. I will.'

'One day, I'll hold you to that.'

We stood and gazed about the island. More bombs fell over Valletta.

One man was admitted to F Block with paralysis of all his limbs and difficulty in breathing. I scanned through Anna's notes, to confirm the diagnosis, but I recognised this disease from the National. I knew immediately that I was examining a case of polio.

Without prompt treatment, the patient would die as he smothered and drowned in his own secretions. The virus was particularly active, injuring and destroying nerve cells that controlled his muscles. The only way to keep him alive was through manual ventilation, pumping his chest by hand.

Quickly, I ripped his shirt open to reveal the thin, malnourished body. I felt for the lower part of the sternum, a sharp edge of bone, automatically measuring two finger widths up. My hands locked, arms straight, I pressed down with the heel of the palm. The chest was compressed before springing back up, dragging air into the weakened lungs. I pressed down again, repeating the action, until tiredness had the better of me. It was exhausting, and Olivia Merciecp took over while I recovered my own breath.

We worked in shifts to keep him alive. Long, endless, shifts. And then another case was admitted, this one struggling to swallow, followed by another one just like the first. They all had difficulty speaking. Our nurses were trained quickly, and we worked together in one continuous rota. It was the only way, and their only chance for survival. I was taking a short, essential, rest when Matron returned to the ward, a stout, red-faced Colonel stumbling alongside her. I recognised the rank from his stripes. She beckoned me to the desk where I performed a weary salute.

'No need for any of that man, sit down.' He gestured to the chair in a voice that was not to be argued with.

'Colonel Winter to see you, Harold. I'll speak to you later.' With a flash of skirt, Matron turned to leave the ward. The Colonel sat opposite me, scraping his chair noisily across the stone floor. He removed his hat to uncover a bald head polished smooth as a bowling ball. He grimaced, revealing a jumble of small, yellow teeth. I glanced towards the patients, to check that everything remained under relative control.

'Sergeant Fisher,' he began, the voice too loud for our proximity, 'I believe you trained at the best neurological hospital back home.'

'That's right, sir,' I looked directly at his round face, the prominent jowled cheeks. His thin lips moved quickly, delivering a fine mist of saliva.

'Good. It turns out you're the only man we've got here with experience of treating polio. We're putting you in charge with immediate effect, and we'll keep all the cases here on F Block. What else will you need?'

'We could do with more help, sir. If we get any more patients we'll be struggling. And we used iron lungs back at the National, sir.'

'I was expecting you to say that.' He smiled so quickly that I wondered if I'd imagined it. 'We've got one on the island. At the naval hospital, Bighi.'

I knew this place. It had been flattened by a bomb.

'Only problem is, it's buried under the ruins. It will need salvage and repair, but we've already got men on the case. Major Merryweather will, of course, assist you. Anything else that you want?'

'What about more antibiotics, sir? For the other patients.'

'I wish I could help you there. This damn siege!' He stood slowly. 'Right then, if that's all I shall be off. Good man, Fisher.' He strolled from the ward in no particular hurry. Olivia Merciecp glanced up and called over, 'Harold, can you help?'

I walked quickly to the patient, well aware that the

powerful stink of sweat I detected was coming from myself. My arms slid over both sides of my body and I wanted to take my shirt off, it was so hot, but this was not allowed. My sleeves were still rolled up and I locked my hands together once again before returning them onto the damp, slippery chest. I pushed down. The patient stared up at me, his gaze beyond the room. I watched his chest inflate with my efforts, concentrating solely on maintaining this task.

When I returned to Mess in the evening, I barely had strength to carry my tray. I tried to pick up a fork, but it was no good; my hands were useless and numb, no longer able to grip. I needed a pal to cut up my food and feed it to me, like a baby. At first, he thought that I was joking.

Rest alone enabled the strength and feeling to return, but there was little time allowed for this. Under my supervision, we now kept six patients alive who were unable to breathe without assistance. We worked all day and all night, interminable, desperate shifts, until the iron lung was finally delivered operable to F Block. To his credit, Colonel Winter supervised it himself.

The Nuffield Drinker iron lung was identical to ones we'd used at the National, except for the obvious signs of salvage. A split had been repaired along the entire right side, resembling a line of untidy sutures. It was badly charred and still retained a scorched odour of burning. But it would make our task much easier, and I was delighted to assist positioning it into the corner of the ground floor ward.

The Drinker consisted of a large airtight chamber into which the patient was slid horizontally. Only the head protruded through a tight rubber seal about the neck. A set of dirty old bellows had been connected, and these could be opened to lower the pressure within the chamber, so causing the chest to expand. Fresh air was drawn into the lungs through the mouth of the patient, with expiration passive. It was far less demanding physically, but the problem was that we had one iron lung and six patients to treat.

Our first admission was placed immediately into the Drinker, and I worked the bellows carefully. The lung wheezed into action, working perfectly, and I thanked the Colonel for delivering it. I explained to my staff the correct speed of operation, and how to position the patient.

Colonel Winter had decided that we should give all cases an equal time in the Drinker, to provide them an equivalent chance of survival. What he failed to take into account was that their conditions varied in severity, and it did not take long before we lost our first two admissions. Many of the men had begun to speak in euphemisms, in an attempt to make our situation appear less real, and I was informed that these two men had "bought it". I couldn't do this, insistent that they report the men had died. But words could not change reality; our situation was getting desperate.

The policy needed changing, and it was now agreed between the Major and myself that only those patients with the best prospects of recovery should be placed in the Drinker. Time was of the essence, and we couldn't go on as before. It was a great idea in theory, but the practice was something else.

Some men wanted to live at any cost. Others craved death, having no wish to remain alive and helpless. These wishes had to be ignored, and I walked methodically around the ward, checking medical charts and readings, selecting who should be placed in the Drinker. It was a hateful responsibility.

The Major joined me on many of these inspections. One

young private, a recent admission, pleaded to be left to die. He said he didn't want his fiancée to see him reduced to a cripple, to have to look after him. The Major picked up the chart at the end of his bed, nodded encouragingly, and turned to me. 'Give him a turn, Fisher.' The patient groaned in dismay, and when I positioned him into the Drinker I was careful to avoid eye contact. I shut my ears to all his protests. Another patient watched this, and later called me over. 'You heartless bastard,' he said. 'If you were any man yourself, you'd let him be.'

Another older man wanted to live, but his prognosis was deemed as poor. 'I'm sorry,' the Major had said, 'got to keep the Drinker free for other cases.' We left him crying with rage, the animal hatred in his eyes terrible to bear.

The number of fatalities crept up as we continued to admit new cases, and I now witnessed many faces of death. There was the weak, the calm acceptance; the fighter, teeth bared, howling for survival; the repentant, the sad, the man who exhaled, 'I've led a wicked life.' It was then that the war found a home inside me, as it had already with Matron. The only choice for self-protection was forcing yourself to become numb and insensitive. You had to learn quickly how to forget.

There were days when I borrowed my calm from the sea, and I could not have coped without the quiet determination of Nan. We met in the shade of the chapel whenever possible, inside the hospital gardens.

'How do you manage to do it?' I asked her. 'I'm sick of watching people die. What's the point in even trying?'

She touched my arm, so gentle, studying me with understanding reflected in those deep dark eyes.

'I know, Harry, but we've got no choice. We've got to

keep going, the patients need us.'

'But I can't even show any emotion. I've got to act strong all the time. It's driving me mad!'

'We'll give each other strength. So long as we have each other, we can do it.' She looked up at the sky, still holding onto my arm. 'It will be dark soon. Come on, let's go to Mdina.'

'So long as we're not too long. I'm on duty again tonight.'

We walked quickly, hand in hand, under a late afternoon sun that bled into the sky, staining the horizon a deep crimson. From the peace of Bastion Square, I looked back at M'tarfa, at the hospital. Darkness had fallen early, a single gash of red visible above the old building.

'Don't think about tomorrow, Harry. Just one day at a time, it's the only way.'

She spoke with absolute certainty, determined to reassure me. I reached out to take hold of her hand.

'I know that you're right. I'm just tired of acting strong, pretending I don't have any feelings. It's getting so bad, Nan, I've even considered smothering patients who don't want to live. I got so far as picking up the pillow with one guy, I'd been thinking about it for hours. He wanted me to do it, and then Matron came into the ward. That was at night, too. I'm getting so messed up now, I'm not sure what's right any more.'

She turned to face me, placing one hand on my neck to stroke my cheek.

'I do understand, it's been tough on Surgical too. But what we're doing is right, Harry. We've got to carry on. You can't go losing it now, who would I have then?'

'What would I do without you?'

'Luckily for you, you'll never need to know.' She bent

forwards and kissed me. 'I'm not going anywhere. And don't you go changing, either. I love the way you are. You're sensitive Harry, that's a good thing.'

She was able to keep me rational, composed, and sane. I worked hard at my duties, attempting to maintain a professional detachment at all times, pretending to be strong for the benefit of the patients. But when I was with Nan, I didn't have to act any more. She allowed me to be myself. I remembered the words of my mother, 'Be careful how you act Harry, or you'll become that person.' It was Nan who kept me from changing. It was Nan who kept me from breaking.

I watched some of our colleagues struggling to cope, even giving in to tears while on duty in the ward. It was the last thing that the patients wanted; they needed to believe in our control, in our faith of their recovery. I was just able to ignore the terrible things that we witnessed daily, to shelve them to one side, and continue with my work. I had Nan to thank for this. She was right, it was the only way to survive.

The outbreak of polio brought with it the greatest number of fatalities experienced on F Block. There was no cure for this disease; we could provide supportive care only, and let it run its course. We did eventually manage to construct basic replicas of the Drinker, through help from the Royal Electrical and Mechanical Engineers. Hand bellows were again provided for when the electricity supply failed, but this was not enough. The big problem that we could not eliminate was deciding on which patients to treat. The continued admission of new cases made sure of this.

To add to our difficulties, a considerable number of the garrison now became scared of contracting this disease. Rumours flew around the island about the severity of the outbreak, exaggerating the extent of its spread, and this led to a new influx of admissions. They suffered from hysterical symptoms only, anxiety neurosis, but still required lumbar puncture and blood counts. We could not spare the time or the materials, and it became a serious problem. Hours of duty increased further, sleep becoming an occasional luxury.

With no supplies reaching the island, we all experienced the bite of hunger. Some of the men bloated up, but I found that my belly gradually disappeared. I was pleased about this, but it didn't stop me from thinking about food. I would be in the middle of a ward round when I would be struck with a sudden craving for bacon and eggs. I would wake up disappointed, in my dream about to tuck into a huge bowl of strawberry ice cream. With Nan, it was Lampuki pie. She explained, in great mouth-watering detail, how this fish was mixed with spinach, cauliflower, chestnuts, and sultanas, and then baked in shortcrust pastry. I'd never tasted it, but felt my own stomach squirm in anticipation. She made it sound so good.

The battle in the sky continued to rage above us, and continued to be one-sided. Our men now had a set amount of ammunition that they were allowed to fire, limited to six rounds per gun per day. It drove the soldiers crazy with frustration; they had to allow the enemy relative freedom to pick us off. The gunpost near Dingli was destroyed, most of the men killed, and it seemed that we were stuck on a road with no way out other than surrender and defeat.

There was one single boost to morale amongst all this desperation, when a consignment of wheat eventually reached the island. It came as no surprise to Nan and me when we were told how it had arrived from nearby Gozo.

'We've got food again, Harry. Did you hear about it?'

A delighted Nan first brought me this news. We stood in

the hospital gardens, looking out towards St. Paul's Bay. She had dried blood crusted onto both sleeves of her shirt. Nan appeared pale, exhausted, but she could not stop herself from smiling.

'I told you it was a good place, didn't I! The farmers have hidden mills, and they shipped it across for us. It must have been so dangerous, with all the mines out there.'

We continued to gaze at the sea. It appeared too pretty, too calm, to be a risk to anyone.

'But aren't they starving too, Nan? How can they spare it?'

'I don't know, but isn't it great news? Food, Harry, we've got food! We'll have to go now, and thank them.'

'When do you think we'll get there, Nan?' I'd asked this question so many times.

'After we've won of course.'

'Will it be long?'

'Not long now, no.'

'I'm glad.'

'Me too.'

We repeated the same conversation, neither of us really believing it, but hoping that if we said it enough times then a germ of truth might spark into life. That it might grow outwards like some beautiful pearl. It never failed to give us hope.

'So how are things in Surgical, Nan?'

'The usual, much the same. And for you?'

'The same, again. We haven't lost anyone today, so that's good.'

The situation did not remain unchanged. While the polio admissions started to decrease, we were hit with a second outbreak of typhoid. Again, sewage had seeped into the water supply.

This time, the men were in no fit state to fight the disease, and four of the initial ten admissions proved fatal. The crisis point killed them quickly. Our recovery rate did improve as we became more expert with the nursing, and when I was able to introduce prophylactic injections. But death could now be seen looking out from the battered, broken windows of F Block.

New admissions were slow to subside. The wards gradually began to resemble their former selves, a few empty beds always available, although the constant clank and wheezing of iron lungs had become a permanent feature of F Block. I still had nights when I was unable to leave my post, and I continued to observe the deaths of men much younger than myself. This didn't get any easier, and it still made no sense at all. Nan was right, it was better this way; I didn't want to understand a world where this was possible. I thought of Overton and Hadley, and all their big talk back in London. If this was their idea of a worthy war, then they could shove it up their arses.

I began the ward round without enthusiasm. It was never good, never easy.

'How are you today, Snailham?'

'Not bad, sir. Hanging in there.'

I reached for his wrist, searching for the thin pulse. A thermometer was placed under the arm, to record his temperature. John Snailham was recovering from typhoid.

'99° now. That's good, soon be down to normal and we can let you go again.'

He smiled. 'But sir, I'm having a rest. Please let me stay a bit longer.'

I moved to the next bed.

'Butterworth, you still in here? How's the leg?'

'A bit sore, sir.' He propped himself up on both elbows.

'Let's have a look, then.' The dressing was stained a fresh yellow, and I sniffed the cloying sweetness of decay. It no longer made me retch. Butterworth was sweating profusely, his sheets drenched, as he continued to run a fever.

'Better get this changed for you.' He rested back onto the bed. 'Sister, this man needs fresh gauze, iodine.'

Olivia Merciecp nodded from behind the desk, struggling to her feet. I knew that she must be as tired and fed up as I was, but she never complained. Not once. I had been lucky to keep the same staff, and they were all excellent nurses. Olivia bustled over to the bed and began to clean the wound. Butterworth was recuperating from a nasty bout of meningitis.

Reaching the far end of the ward, I paused briefly, out of sight of the patients. I was exhausted, in need of a break, and steadied myself at the foot of the stairs. One hand rested against the limestone wall, and I inspected the pale ghostly imprint. It did not resemble any part of my body, coated in fine white icing. It was a wonder that the block was still standing, it shed so much of the damned dust.

I began to climb the steps, one hand reaching instinctively for Dot's bear. He had served me well in some ways, and I hoped that this would continue. The air was cooler on the staircase, a breeze rushed against my face, and I looked forward to finishing this inspection. I hoped I'd be able to sleep, if it wasn't possible to meet with Nan.

Entering the second ward, I knew immediately that something was wrong. We should have had six patients; somebody was missing. I scanned the room, checking for empty beds - it was Gregory who had vanished.

A stumbling noise came from behind me, from the

direction of the balcony. I turned quickly, suddenly worried, and then I saw him appear from out of the gloom, standing some twenty yards in front of me. Gregory had managed to climb onto the stone wall, despite the sling on his arm. He balanced precariously on the thin ledge, swaying gently backwards and forwards. His arms rose and fell like wings.

I had seen this before, when a man gives up hope. I didn't shout, but started to jog towards him, attempting to make little noise. I knew that I could save him, if only he chose to listen. His condition was definitely improving.

I had nearly reached Gregory when he saw me. He shook his head sadly, and mouthed the word 'no'. I noticed the broken front tooth, the stitched forehead. His eyes opened wide and, twisting, he fell backwards. I lunged towards him, grabbing desperately, my fingers brushing against the hairs of his leg. I threw myself against the stone, bending over the edge just in time to watch the smile appear on his face.

I heard the sound, of egg-shell cracking, when his skull split open on the path below. I closed my eyes, gripping the balcony hard until pain in the fingers registered. Another death. Another wasted life. Nan had said that Malta used to be called the nurse of the Mediterranean. It was becoming much more like the curse. I slumped against the stonework. I closed my eyes.

CHAPTER TWELVE

Attack after attack brought about an inevitable erosion of spirit on the island. Of course, it did not help that we were all hungry. Colonel Winter himself had complained of stomach pains, which no medicine could help alleviate. Everybody now carried that familiar, weary look I had first noticed during the Blitz, all eyes dulled and discouraged. People spoke in muted voices. Everybody had a story of heartbreak and loss to relate.

I recall a hard, painful, knot in my stomach, sometimes present for days, and how everything began to appear unreal. Faces appeared magnified and grotesque, the iron lung sound on the ward muffled as if underwater. Time would sometimes slow down, and walking across F Block acquired a semblance of floating. I was not aware of my feet touching the hard stone of the floor. I could not allow myself to relax, to unwind, and if you were unable to dull your senses, you simply broke. Our psychiatric wards provided ample proof of this.

War continued to rage about us, above us. What memories remained took on the quality of visions, and I breathed these in and out. I could not stop them. I recalled individual faces of German pilots flying low over the hospital grounds; the sight of a hospital colleague blown literally into pieces. His body spilt outwards like the Opera House in Valletta, like the door and windows of F Block. I remembered an attack while attending one of countless burials, and watching the coffin bottom open to drop the corpse into a shallow, dusty grave. It made a dreadful thudding sound. The casket would have to be used again.

Sleep became essential and terrible. I attempted to dream of snow, and the silence that could come with it, but this proved futile. My Park Street nightmare resurfaced, now in the company of ugly siblings. Too many images and half-remembered thoughts flooded the scenes, and I often woke up shouting. I was not alone. The worst nightmare had me on an athletics track, under heavy enemy fire. Guns blazed and the men around me were picked off individually until only myself and one other remained. A woman. We aimed at each other from close distance, our guns repeatedly jamming. It was at the very moment that I knew I was about to be shot when my gun exploded into life. The bullet ripped a path through her stomach and she fell. Dead. In this dream, the woman was invariably Gwen.

From the hospital rooftop, I watched more of our planes destroyed on the ground at Ta Qali. This had become a common sight, another incident that required our acceptance. It did not help to let it get to you in any way. Tiredness caused me a permanent headache, and I forgot what it was like to be without hunger. Some of the Maltese farmers began sleeping in fields armed with shotguns, to protect their meagre crop. Soldiers were now being admitted to Surgical for removal of the pellets. I understood quickly that men in prolonged battle were not normal, but changed. It was inevitable.

The constant activity on F Block was interrupted by one thing only, and that was the radio. If at all possible, nursing duties came to a standstill in order to listen to the broadcasts of Winston Churchill.

The wireless, large and cumbersome, was positioned in the centre of the desk, and I cranked up the volume so that everybody could listen. The staff collected near me, at the far end of the ward, and I surveyed the ward to notice the row of faces twisting and craning towards us, feeding off the words like baby birds.

A deliberate pause between sentences made Churchill the complete spellbinder. We trusted and believed in him. We needed him. Heads nodded in earnest agreement to his speeches, eyes became more animated; his words provided a source of courage and inspiration, possessing tremendous power, to keep our hope alive at a time when victory seemed impossible. Still, no convoys had been able to reach us, but the atmosphere in F Block was always lightened, more optimistic, after these missives.

I left the wireless on for the broadcasts of Miss Vera Lynn. They were just as good for the patients as Churchill's, the messages conveyed in her songs boosting morale through reminding people of home. It came as a surprise that it was always London I thought and dreamed of, never Folkestone, although I could easily imagine never walking in St. James Park or Whitechapel Road again. But with Nan, here on Malta, I did not want to be anywhere else.

We continued to meet whenever possible, but nursing duties limited such opportunities. Our time spent together provided more strength and comfort than any radio broadcast could offer, and an agreement had been reached between us. The walk to Buskett Gardens and Dingli took too long now; there was never sufficient time. Mdina was much closer, and still sometimes possible to reach. Leaving M'tarfa, when you climbed the track that sloped up to the silent city, the second tall palm tree on the right led into a field. It was far enough from barracks to offer some privacy and we chose to meet here. Hidden behind the ancient hibiscus and oleander trees.

I liked to come at night, always unsure if Nan was going

to be able to make it. It was never cold, and I stripped down to my underpants, lying on top of my clothes. The earth was flat in this spot, and the dust soon brushed clean from my uniform. I rested back and watched the sky fill with warm, white stars, lulled by the song of cicadas. A perfume from nearby flowers touched the air, washing over my skin, and this was far preferable to the staleness of barracks. Sometimes, I fell asleep.

Nan, if she arrived, would undress and lie down beside me. I would gradually become aware of her presence, turning slowly, in fear of disturbing a dream and causing her disappearance. Our lips would meet first, followed by arms, and then what was left of our stomachs.

'I've missed you.' Nan's opening words never changed. 'Do you know how much I love you?'

'How much?'

'Too much.'

'Well I love you more!'

She smiled, and punched my arm.

'You can't! It's not possible.'

We came together and the war ceased to exist. For a few hours, nothing else was solid or real. Stars beat and pulsed in the night sky, illuminating our naked bodies. Those few stolen hours became priceless, my single motivation to keep on breathing. They became my iron lung.

Major Merryweather entered F Block earlier than usual. He looked agitated or excited, I couldn't tell, changed from his usual calm manner. The polio and typhoid outbreaks appeared to be on the decline, and I wondered what troubled him. He caught me looking and beckoned towards the desk.

'Got some news today, Fisher, thought you'd like to

know.' He spoke quietly, in order that no one else could hear.

'What is it, Major?'

'It's just a whisper, so keep it to yourself, but I hear that help is on its way.'

'Are you sure?' I spoke too loud and he shushed me, irritated. I'd become so used to the siege that it was hard to imagine anything could change. It was impossible to envisage an end to it all.

'Quiet, man. Don't want to get the patients excited. But we should have some more Spitfires soon, you'll see. And they've finally changed the policy at Ta Qali, got better organised at last. We shouldn't be losing so many planes in future. I think this could be it Fisher.' He placed one hand on my shoulder, uncharacteristically informal. 'A change in fortune, at last!'

'Really, Major?'

'Yes. Things might finally be on the up. I wanted you to know, but make sure you keep it to yourself. Now I'm off to tell Matron, I'll be back in half an hour.'

He walked quickly from the building while I remained at the desk. It just didn't seem possible that help could ever reach us. It was the ninth consecutive month that we had found ourselves under constant attack, with no sign of the action reducing. Of course it would be good if the situation were to improve, but a new worry concerned me. Anna McHardy had been moved on, transferred to Egypt. If I wasn't needed on the island, could the same thing happen to me? I resolved not to think about this. It was daft - there were enough things going on that required my attention without having to make stuff up.

The Major had told me not to share this information, but there was no way I was hiding anything from Nan. After what had happened about Gwen, I'd promised never to withhold anything from her again. The only thing was, this time, I didn't get a chance to tell her.

Two days later, and two nights without Nan, it was a strange-looking Matron who rushed into F Block. She nearly ran across the ward, against all the rules, smiling as if she'd just got back from sliding along a rainbow after finding her pot of gold. For a second I thought she had cracked, but there was no mistaking her genuine joy.

'Harold! Harold! Have you heard?'

I stood up from my bedside inspection; Butterworth would soon be discharged, his temperature had at last returned to normal. He had been telling me about his family, and how he intended to take up diving as soon as his health was improved.

'What is it Matron?' She rushed across the ward, grabbing hold of my hands. 'What's happened?'

'Wonderful news, Harold. A convoy has managed to reach us. We'll have supplies again!'

The Major had not been wrong.

'When did it get here?' It was Butterworth who spoke, attempting to climb out of bed. I had to take hold of his arm; he wasn't strong enough for this yet.

'Just now. I've just been told about it.'

An American oil tanker, *Ohio*, had apparently managed to crawl into the harbour at Valletta, her decks nearly awash. She was in a bad way after an enemy dive-bomber had crashed on board. One bomb had exploded in the engine room, but most of the cargo remained intact. *Ohio* had been unloaded as quickly as possible, and we now had supplies to keep us going a little longer. We not only had food, but also fuel and ammunition. Finally, we would be able to fight back.

I managed to reach our meeting place that evening, where Nan already sat waiting. When I ducked behind the hibiscus, she jumped to her feet, delighted.

'Oh Harry, isn't it wonderful!'

She threw herself against me, demanding to be kissed.

'I know. It hasn't really sunk in yet. I wonder what it will mean?'

'It means that we'll win!' She kissed me again, our teeth cracking together. 'You know what day it is, don't you?'

'What do you mean, Nan?'

'It's the 15th August. The feast of Santa Maria. This is no coincidence, Harry, this is God's work. That ship should never have reached us, you know a bomb went off on board?' I nodded. 'I tell you, it means we're going to win! Now hurry up and love me, will you?' She grabbed at my shirt with both hands, the buttons popping open. 'I've missed you. Do you know how much I love you?'

From the roof of the hospital, a new consignment of Spitfires was spotted at Ta Qali. Now, when the air raid siren sounded, we watched as they were mobilised rapidly, taking off unarmed if necessary, and disappearing into the blue. The pilots flew low over the sea until the attack had petered away, so avoiding early destruction. Afterwards, the planes were armed as quickly as possible.

Four other merchantman boats had survived the voyage with *Ohio*, and in the following months further supplies were able to reach the island. By November, the siege was effectively over. A tidal wave of optimism swept across Malta; we believed that if we could survive that, we could survive anything.

The escorting aircraft carriers transported more Spitfires

to the island, replacing all the planes that we had witnessed destroyed. Increasing numbers of people now chose to ignore the air raid sirens and shelters, preferring to continue with their work and watch the action in the sky. Whenever possible, I resumed my position on top of the operating theatre.

It was immediately obvious that the Spitfires possessed superior manoeuvrability, and I witnessed our pilots reap a rich harvest of enemy planes. Aircraft exploded in blinding flashes of light before plummeting out of the sky. I saw aircrew from opposing sides shoot at each other while they floated down to the ground, their screams cutting the air. The occupants of crashed and burning enemy planes were jeered to their deaths, accompanied with shouts of 'let the bastards burn.' There were never offers of help. Buried savagery and raw anger had risen to the surface, dazzling in their eyes. These men were not themselves; you cannot live through such events without change, it is impossible. War brought out the best and worst in men and women. I noticed this every day.

The Italian and German pilots began to jettison their bombs quickly and haphazardly, no longer darting in close, reluctant to enter into a dogfight. Injuries and damage on the island were substantially reduced, convoys continued to reach us, and it seemed that the tide had definitely turned. Finally, we could believe Churchill's victory was possible.

It was unusual to be summoned by Matron to the Major's office in the hospital, for I was expecting his arrival on the ward. I climbed to the second floor of the building wondering what was up, and turned left as instructed to reach his room. It was a further surprise to discover that this was small and dark, more of a cupboard than an office, after the relative grandeur of Sliema. The door stood open and Major Merryweather crouched low, his back towards me. He was searching for a book on one of his shelves, and I tapped lightly onto the door.

'Come in.' He stood and turned quickly. 'Harold, you got my message.' The Major took my hand in his own, shaking it warmly. I felt uncomfortable - he never called me this. 'More good news, man. I didn't want to broadcast it on the ward.'

'What is it, sir?'

'Sit down. Sit down.' He smiled, removing his spectacles. The Major wiped the back of one hand across his forehead, dislodging pearly beads of sweat that splashed onto the floor. The hair above his ears looked greyer each time that I saw him. There was only one chair in the room.

'I'm all right standing, thank you.'

'As you will. As you will.' He sat himself, replacing the spectacles, and smiled. 'Your work has been recognised by Colonel Winter. He thanked me, but I told him he should speak to you in person. He said there wasn't time. Anyway, they want to offer you a promotion.' The Major spoke rapidly, his words running into each other.

I took a step towards him, listening carefully.

'A position has come up in Algiers. Far more prestigious. What do you think?'

'I don't want it, sir.' I spoke too quickly.

'Why not, man? It's a good offer for you.' He frowned.

'I don't want to leave, sir. I feel useful on F Block. What about with the polio outbreak - I was the only one with any experience. Who would take my place?'

'And this wouldn't have anything to do with your Maltese girlfriend, would it?' He leaned towards me, speaking slowly now. I swallowed hard, amazed that he should know about

Nan. Matron must have told him.

'No, sir. Not at all.'

'I hope not, Fisher.' He studied me intently. 'You can't let that sway you. We've a war to fight, remember?'

'Yes, sir. I know, sir.'

'Well all right. I shall let him know your answer. I didn't want to lose you, anyway. Better get back to work then.'

I was dismissed and he resumed the search for his book. There was no way that I would ever volunteer to leave Nan, but I felt real concern that I'd nearly had no choice in the matter. It made another outbreak of disease appear almost desirable if this should keep me on the island, and my heart raced like wind in a storm. It had been another close call. I touched Dot's bear in my pocket and said 'thank you' one more time.

The day passed in a blur. I couldn't stop thinking about the offer of promotion, and how lost I should have been if ordered to leave the island. It was a terrible prospect. I tried to carry on with work as normal, but Olivia Merciecp noticed that something was wrong. 'Is there anything I can do to help?' she had whispered quickly during the ward round.

I managed to leave F Block on time, and was delighted to spot Nan ahead of me. She was walking out of the hospital gardens. I called her name and sprinted between the trees, past the chapel, to reach her side. Fierce heat remained in the day, no wind to cool us down, and already I was sweating.

'Are you finished as well?'

She waited outside the gates.

'Yes, Harry, I got off earlier than usual. It was a little quieter today.' Nan brushed the dust from my shirt, and I noticed the angry red mark above her left eye. I bent to kiss this instinctively.

'How did it happen?'

She sighed, reaching to touch the affected area. 'This morning, Harry, I felt that something wasn't right - you know that feeling, when something is on your mind, and you can't work out what it is? Anyway, I wasn't paying enough attention and hit my head on a cupboard. It was me who'd left it open. What an idiot!'

'Poor you.' I took her hand. 'So what do you want to do now?'

'Shall we walk to Buskett then?' It had been months since we had managed to visit the gardens.

'You're on!'

We set out straight away, without bothering to change from our uniforms, sharp orange sunlight burning onto our faces. I wanted to put a needle into the day, to bleed the heat out, but Nan seemed unaffected.

Before anything, I had to tell her about the Major, it continued to trouble me badly. I hurried an explanation while she looked worried, shaking her head. Her mouth turned down in a frown.

'So they nearly took you away from me, Harry? I don't like that.' The words came thick as tar, 'What would I have done then?'

'What about me? I don't want to go. But they didn't, did they? We're still here.' I squeezed her hand, pulling her into a hug. 'They can't separate us that easily.'

We resumed our walk, but Nan remained silent. She continued to frown.

'Hey, you! Cheer up! Live in the present, remember? We're off to Buskett Gardens, both finished our work, just the two of us. That's got to be good, hasn't it?' I protested.

'You're right, I know, but it's such a horrible thought.'

'I know.'

Evidence of war had disfigured the land since our last visit. Old stone walls and farmhouses had been flattened after long years spent undisturbed; the field where I had stolen grapes was now reduced to a large, ugly crater. I knew that Nan would have noticed this, and attempted to distract her.

'Nan, do you know how much I love you?' She turned to look at me, managing a thin smile. 'I'm not going anywhere.'

'So how much do you love me, Harry?'

'More than you love me!'

'Impossible.' She broke away. 'Come on, I'll race you to the gardens.'

I let her win. It was too good a sight to remain behind her, watching her. We stopped at the gates of the Verdala Palace and we kissed, a good, hard, kiss.

'Do you know what this is now?' She gestured to the building. 'A school for refugees. Their homes have all been destroyed.'

We kissed again, more slowly. I was even hotter now. 'Nan, do you fancy a swim? It's been ages, hasn't it?'

'Yes, let's do that first.'

We walked the remaining part of the journey hand in hand. Nan led the way down the path on the cliff, near the Magdalena chapel, and quickly we were in the water. It felt glorious. I watched her shrink into the distance; she was a much stronger swimmer than me, while I was happy to float on my back.

The sky was a perfect blue. Again, there was not a cloud in sight, and I was comparing this to the grimy sky over London when a hand grabbed through my legs, taking me by surprise. My head went under the water, salt stinging into my eyes. When I resurfaced, Nan was choking with laughter beside me.

'Got you,' she spluttered.

'And now, I'm going to get you!'

I splashed towards her. She made no attempt to escape. My hands locked onto her shoulders, I was going to duck her under the water, but the touch of her skin changed my mind. I kissed the side of her neck, savouring the taste in my mouth. Her hands reached around me, taking hold of my buttocks, pulling me into her.

We struggled to the shallow water, Nan now on top, lowering herself onto me. I began to move inside her. Sea and blue sky swam before my eyes, cliffs the colour of honey, and then I heard the noise.

'What's that, Nan?'

'What?'

'Can't you hear it?'

She stopped moving. The droning grew louder. It was a plane. I looked above her shoulder and saw the dark spot on the horizon. It was definitely getting closer.

'Ignore it, Harry.' She lifted above me, then downwards. 'Ignore it.'

I tried, but the noise was becoming louder.

'Nan, wait.'

She held her arms around my neck, now still. I shimmied my body through 90 degrees so that we could both watch the aircraft. It had been aiming towards Fifla but changed direction, veering directly towards us. The noise grew even louder when it began to descend.

'I love you, Harry, you know that,' Nan breathed in my ear with sudden urgency.

The pilot must have spotted us; there was definitely no

mistake. He aimed straight for our heads.

'I love you too, Nan.'

I shut my eyes. The sound grew deafening and I held her tightly, just one thought in my mind. This wasn't such a bad way to go, as naked as my birth, a beautiful woman in my arms. I waited, resigned for the inevitable, but there were no sounds of gunshot when the plane sped low above us.

'Did you see that?' she spoke in amazement.

'See what?'

'He was waving at us. The pilot waved at us.'

I turned to follow the sound. The plane was curving in the blue sky, coming back a second time.

'Watch Harry, it's okay!'

We did not move. The German pilot flew low over the sea, following the line of the cliffs, and this time I kept my eyes open. He was waving, Nan was right, and grinning, too. Before the plane flew over our heads, he stuck one thumb up into the air, and then changed direction for Italy. We watched him recede quickly into the distance.

'I can't believe it, Nan.'

'Me, too,' she laughed.

'Amazing.'

I struggled from beneath her, stumbling over stones to reach the shore.

'Harry, where are you going?'

'To Buskett Gardens, it's safer.' I rushed to put on some clothes, underpants crumpled into the pocket of my shorts, before passing Nan her uniform.

The road was empty. We ran, laughing, along the dusty path that led between the trees. It was cooler here, silent, and our feet crunched loudly on the dry earth. I kept hold of Nan's hand, urgent, leading her to the site of the twisted vine.

Clothes were discarded onto the ground and I threw my body decadently onto the top of them. I watched as Nan undressed before positioning herself over my stomach. Anything was now possible. Nothing was written in stone. Familiar words danced loud in my head; nothing could go wrong, nothing would go wrong. For a while, we were able to love undisturbed.

CHAPTER THIRTEEN

After the siege of the island, I suffered from constant tiredness. It felt as if I should never be allowed to sleep properly again, and even when an opportunity arose, I woke at regular intervals. My subconscious was always busy, anticipating the next air raid and its siren, preparing my body for the run to the hospital. This was nothing unusual; everybody I knew suffered the same way.

I then began to pass some half pint of bright red arterial blood with moderate frequency. I chose to ignore this too, believing my insides had simply lost a routine, it would soon sort itself out. It was only after collapsing with dizziness, halfway along St. David's Road on the way to work, that I placed myself on sick parade. I was reluctant to leave my post, well aware that my experience could be needed at any time.

It was somewhat ironic that I ended up an admission in F Block, on the upstairs ward, where the Regimental Medical Officer performed a cursory examination. A small brute of a man, his single heavy eyebrow knotted in concentration while stubby fingers jabbed and poked into my abdomen. He hurt me, grunting with disapproval if I should involuntarily let out a groan. 'Better get the Major to see you, Fisher,' were the only words that he spoke.

I lay staring at the ceiling, cursing this state of affairs, when it suddenly dawned on me that I'd been placed in Gregory's old bed. 'Shit,' I muttered under my breath, staring at the dark yellow stain on the limestone above my head. We had a leak coming in from somewhere.

Major Merryweather expressed surprise on discovering

the identity of his patient.

'Bloody hell Fisher, what's happened to you?'

Unlike most of the men, I'd never heard him swear before. The words jarred in my ears, made worse through unfamiliarity. Briefly, I explained the medical history.

'You bloody fool!' he exploded. 'Thought you of all people would have known better. We need you fit and well, haven't got time to have you off ill.'

'Yes, sir. I realise that.'

'Well why didn't you say anything? I've seen you enough times, it's not like you haven't had a chance.'

'I didn't want to bother you, sir. I thought it would get better.'

'You thought, did you? Well we all know what thought did!' He whipped back the sheet in an angry flourish. 'Let's have a look at you, then.'

His hands reached for the right side of my stomach, just above the liver, immediately targeting the source of the problem. He pressed down firmly and I grimaced in shock, a sharp pain radiating outwards. White light flashed behind my eyes. The Major continued this inspection, his hands expert in their investigation.

'Well you can probably tell me what the problem is, Fisher?' I shook my head, resting back on the thin pillow. 'I think you've got a case of chronic amoebiasis and hepatitis. We'll get stool and blood samples off to the lab and keep you in here. I still think you're a fool to leave it this long!'

The rage in which he spoke caused the RMO to raise his solitary eyebrow, a sardonic smirk appearing on his already ugly face.

'I'm sorry, Major.' I felt that I'd let everyone down, particularly myself, but Major Merryweather was careful to pat me on the shoulder before leaving the ward. He removed his glasses and wiped a palm across his brow. He looked exhausted.

'We'll soon get you right, Harold.' This time, he spoke with concern.

Appropriate samples were despatched and confirmation quickly confirmed. I had an ulcerated colon and gross inflammation of the liver. Treatment necessitated the procedure of sigmoidoscopy, and to my horror I knew exactly what this entailed.

A sigmoidoscope consists of a long, small-bored, hollow metal tube coupled with a blunt rounded end on a rod. The rod is withdrawn as soon as the instrument has entered the rectum, and a light is then positioned at the end of the tube for illumination. Passage into the colon is aided by pumping in air. The procedure is supposedly only painful when the colon is inflamed or ulcerated - mine, of course, was both. When Major Merryweather returned to the bedside, he look suitably grim-faced.

'Well Fisher, are you ready then?'

'As I'll ever be, sir.' It was a pretence of joviality.

Squatting on elbows and knees, I was instructed in no uncertain terms to raise my arse high into the air. Merryweather attempted to insert the damn thing into me, but it was to no avail. I remembered the patient who had complained it was like having a burning bush shoved up his rear end; I'd thought at the time he must have been exaggerating, but not while I struggled to climb from the bed.

To my dismay, the Major called for the RMO to have a go, who was known for his aggressive technique. Again, I tried to haul myself off the bed whilst the two of them pulled me backwards and onto the instrument. I put up a good fight, connecting with one particularly well-aimed kick onto the chest of the RMO, but this only seemed to encourage him. With one sharp push, they had the thing inside me and I howled in severe pain. It hurt like sheer bloody hell.

The investigation revealed widespread areas of ulceration, and blood loss had occurred through damage to these by hard motions. Unfortunately for me, treatment was as unpleasant as the disease.

Six injections of emetine were required, causing profound nausea, followed by seven quinoxyl enemas. The foot of the bed was raised in order to run this fluid directly into my rectum, where it was to be retained for as long as possible. I had always suffered a predisposition for wind, but to fart now would have been disastrous. I hadn't seen Nan since my admission to the ward, but made Sister Merciecp promise that she would not allow her to see me in this position. It was bad enough that it was in front of my own staff, and I wondered if they should ever be able to respect me again.

An arsenical preparation of stovarsol followed, together with capsules to be swallowed at night. These contained a mixture of emetine, bismuth, and iodine, ensuring that I felt just as bloody awful as before the treatment had started.

Major Merryweather arrived to check on my progress, walking quickly up the stairs and across the ward.

'How are you doing then, Harold?'

I could tell immediately he was in a good mood through the use of my first name.

'I've felt better, sir.'

'Yes, I'm sure you have. Wouldn't care to swap places, but there you go.' He checked my pulse and temperature. 'Well, we're going to move you, my man. Get you out of here for once, to recuperate and get your strength back.'

I felt a momentary panic; I still hadn't managed to see Nan, and wanted to let her know what was happening.

'Where am I going, Major?'

'A place called Marsaxlokk. It's on the east coast of the island.'

I felt an instant fluttering in my stomach. Marsaxlokk. This had to be another good omen. Marsaxlokk was Nan's home town.

She came to visit me in the evening still dressed in army uniform, her face pale and drawn with worry.

'Oh Harry, I've only just found out where you were. I've been going to the field and wondered what had stopped you.' She reached to hold my hand, planting a kiss in the centre of my forehead. 'It's not like you not to show up.'

'I've missed you, Nan. There was no way I could tell you where I was.'

She fought to hold back tears. 'You! You look beat, Harry. What's happened? Olivia just caught me, to tell me you'd been admitted.'

I explained the symptoms and diagnosis, what they had done with me.

'But you never told me, Harry! I thought we had a deal.'

'Sorry. I thought that it was nothing, I didn't want to worry you.'

'Nothing! It doesn't look like that from where I'm standing.'

'Please Nan, the Major's already had a go. Sit down.' I patted the bed. 'Here, next to me.'

Nan looked exhausted, her movements slower, more awkward, than usual. I rested one hand on her leg.

'You see?' I smiled for her benefit. 'I'm feeling better

already. So how's it been on Surgical?'

'Better than it was. But I feel beat today, and now I find out about you.' She placed one hand on my own. 'It's not good.'

'Well you know what we need to do, then?' I struggled to sit upright.

'What's that?'

'Take a trip to Gozo!'

'Just tell me when, Harry. Tell me when. And you lie back again, I can see you're not well.'

'Only after you've kissed me.'

She glanced about the room. It was quiet on the ward, all the other patients apparently sleeping or reading. She kissed me quickly, on the lips.

'You'll never guess where they're sending me, Nan?'

'I'm too tired to guess. I've no idea.'

'Marsaxlokk! I'll be able to meet your family.'

'Maybe. Yes.' Nan's tears finally broke free. 'Just you get yourself better.'

'Will you come and visit me?'

'I'll come as often as I can. You know that.'

In the morning, I was transferred into the back of an old army van. There was no window, and the only thing I could ascertain on the drive to Marsaxlokk was that the roads were in a bad way. And that it was hot. My back and sides hurt from repeated bouncing on the hard wooden bench seat.

I was aware of the van climbing, struggling up a hill, before finally coming to a halt. The driver hopped from the cab and flung open the back doors, helping me out into brilliant white sunlight. The air smelt so different, so clean.

We stood on a rise overlooking the sea. In front of us, a vivid blue saltwater scar divided two headlands that poked fingers out into the bay.

'Delimara Point, mate. Your new home.'

'I thought I was going to Marsaxlokk?'

'You're here, mate. Look over there.' He pointed to a jumble of little houses dotted around a tiny harbour. Colourful fishing boats jigged up and down amidst the rapid sparkle of water. 'That's Marsaxlokk.'

I turned to look at the house. It was big, a plain affair of grey stone and flat roof, with three large windows positioned at the front. It was situated three terraces up from the bay, and two other villas were located nearby. They all appeared to be identical.

'Should be quiet here, mate.' The driver continued to speak. 'There's a gunpost at the end of the Point, but out of sight is out of mind. That's what I always say. Come on, I'll help you inside.'

I was escorted into a large room where six beds stood arranged in military precision. Two of them were occupied, their inhabitants asleep and snoring. It was bright and pleasant, thanks to the big windows, and smelled fresh, thankfully free of the cling of carbolic acid.

'So which bed do you want, mate?'

'He's having the one nearest the door, thank you.' We both turned to identify the source of this formidable voice. A tiny Maltese woman clip-clopped briskly across the tiled floor. Her white dress was spotless, and not one single black hair on her head dared to stray out of place. It was tied back, sensible, severe.

'I am Nurse Vella, and this will be Harold Fisher, yes?'

I nodded. She was plump and only marginally less fearsome close up. 'Thank you driver, you may go now.'

He saluted and disappeared, obviously pleased to make

his escape. 'See you later mate, hope you're better soon,' he called from the door.

'Thanks for the lift.'

Nurse Vella was glaring with hands held on hips, impatient, and I stood facing her, unsure what was expected of me.

'What are you waiting for, Fisher? Get into bed then, I've got other jobs to be doing than you.'

'But surely the fresh air might do me some good?' I pleaded. She made me want to return outside as quickly as possible.

'Yes, tomorrow it might!'

She watched me undress to my underpants before helping me climb onto the bed. A white gown was found from somewhere, and my first day in Marsaxlokk was spent waiting. I waited to be allowed in the sunshine, to sit outside looking over the bay. I waited to get better, and I waited for Nan to arrive. I had time on my hands, and for the first occasion in a long while, I considered my previous life. The one I had left behind. On that first day in Marsaxlokk, I didn't want to but I thought about Gwen.

After Gwen's return to London, we moved quickly to Marchmont Street. It was easy to find property at this time, with many people now choosing to move to supposedly safer towns in the country, and rent was cheaper than at Elsham Road. I didn't want to leave the Marriotts, but staying with them in Hackney was obviously not an option. With Marchmont Street, at least I was moving to a familiar part of the city. I still had friends at the National, the British Museum was two minutes walk away, and the cycle ride to work was considerably reduced. I decided to make a go of it, to find out what was left of our relationship.

The flat was small but comfortable, situated on the first floor above a café. The living room, overlooking the street, was painted a warm orange colour, and previous tenants had left prints of Africa hanging on the walls. All of the furniture was constructed from a dark wood; the display cabinet, dining table, and chairs. It had a striking, foreign feel that I liked. We had one dark red bedroom, the bed smaller than at Elsham Road, its mattress lumpy and edged with hard springs. Kitchen and bathroom were adequate. Neither of us was interested in cooking, and it was possible to eat in the café downstairs, to supplement our food rations. We both put on a show of excitement at the prospect of our new home, a fresh start, but there remained a definite awkwardness between Gwen and myself. I found that I now missed Diana, for she at least provided some distraction. Her lively presence made it less obvious that our relationship now floundered, struggling to breathe.

Each morning, we were woken punctually by the rehearsals of a tenor who lived a few doors along the street. I never saw him, but he must surely have been a professional opera singer, his voice rich and smooth as fine brandy. It made a vast improvement from my battered old tin alarm clock, and I often rose early just to listen to his songs. I then grabbed my bicycle for work, leaving Gwen in bed to whatever she did with her days. I knew she had begun to socialise with some of the other tenants, and when I arrived home in the evenings I watched her becoming visibly happier. She would sing quietly to herself, tending a line of red geraniums that grew in the window box outside the kitchen. We shared a bed again, but there was no subsequent improvement in our relationship.

News from the war fought overseas was bad and getting worse, and we listened in dismay to Hitler's relentless advance. My own work at the hospital was proving easier than previous training, and life quickly reverted to the monotony of one long routine. This didn't agree with me at all; I felt that I could and should be doing more, that something important was missing. I wanted to escape already from my new life with Gwen, but this involved not only running away. I needed somewhere to arrive. When the call for National Service arrived, I was delighted; war seemed to provide the answer.

'I think I'm going to sign up,' I said to Gwen.

She made no attempt to stop me.

'Which part, Harold?' She walked out of the living room and into the kitchen. I heard the splashing of a tap.

'The Navy. You know I've always loved the sea. Thought I'd try my luck on a boat.'

'I don't think that's such a good idea.' She returned to the room with a glass of water in her hand, before sitting opposite me at the table.

'Why not?'

'One of my hunches. I think you should join the Army.'

'But I don't really want to, I fancy the Navy.'

'Join the Army, Harold. I'm telling you, you'll have a better chance of survival. You know I'm usually right.'

It was true. Premonitions and coincidence had become a frequent occurrence in our life together, with Gwen's hunches usually proving correct. I let her sway me once again, making the decision for me, with the one consolation that I would be following in my father's footsteps. At least he would be pleased. The wait for conscription began.

Spring had arrived when Gwen informed me how she had

bumped into an old friend in St. James Park. We sat in the café downstairs over plates of egg and chips, and there was something clinical, detached, in her manner that made me take extra notice. I stopped eating, taking a swig of hot, milky tea, from a mug that still tasted of soap. Gwen chose her words with a calculated precision. She spoke with halting pauses, unusually hesitant, like a bad actress repeating lines that somebody else had written for her.

'Fred works in the Civil Service. We got talking about when you join the Army and leave, Harold. I told him I didn't know what I would do. Where I would live. He said that I could stay with his family.'

'But you hardly know him.' I stared through the grease of the window at rain that fell heavily from a dirty grey sky. It ran streaming across the pavement, delivering all discarded rubbish into the gutter. A crumpled old cigarette packet washed over the edge, disappearing from sight, followed by sweet wrappers. I had been led to believe that Fred was merely an acquaintance, not even a friend. I had certainly never met him. 'What about his wife?' I asked. 'Is he married? Does she agree to this?'

'Just think about it, will you? It makes sense. I don't want to be left on my own, you know that. I thought that you cared about me.' Her voice remained altered, aloof.

'I do.' She made it difficult to argue. 'But doesn't it seem a bit sudden? I'd like to know who he is, for a start.'

'You will, Harold. You will.' I felt certain that I detected smugness. 'I don't know his wife, but Fred says she'll be glad of the company. I'm sure that you'll like them both. He says that we can move in straight away, to get settled before you leave.'

I noticed the flush on her usually pale cheeks. It appeared

that everything had been decided, just like the previous move to Marchmont Street, and Gwen's asking for my approval was no more than going through the motions. When I had talked about joining the Services, this concern had never been voiced.

'So how much will it cost us?' I spoke with resignation. There was no real point in arguing, I'd only lose as usual.

'We'll pay exactly the same as here. The only extra will be for food and drink, we'll keep all that separate.' She smiled, triumphant. Gwen returned to her food, no longer interested in me.

I agreed to this plan with reluctance. My hands felt tied. I could find no good reason to decline, especially when I would soon be going away, but I instinctively knew it to be a mistake. That night, my old dream from Park Street returned, an unmistakable bad omen.

We moved to a big semi-detached house in Harrow, at the top of a long winding road. It overlooked parkland at the back, and had four bedrooms, much grander than the Marchmont Street flat.

Fred came running out of the front door to meet us, with effeminate, mincing steps. 'Gwen,' he cried out, 'you've made it,' before kissing her on both cheeks. He shook my hand as an afterthought, and ushered us into the house. He was a short, bespectacled man, who flaunted an extravagant wing-commander style moustache despite never having served in the forces himself. Some problem with his feet, never specified, was offered as the reason for this exclusion. Of course he wanted to sign up, but the damn boys upstairs wouldn't let him. He had fine, foppish, blond hair, flicked constantly from his forehead with tiny, delicate fingers. He stank of cologne, an acrid perfume, which within five minutes of meeting he bragged was shipped over from Paris. I wondered as to Gwen's fondness - there seemed nothing obvious about him to like.

Marjory, Fred's wife, was making pastry in the kitchen. Now she was an altogether different prospect, tall and glamorous despite the flour stuck up to her elbows. She had large brown eyes, a wide mouth with attractively full lips, and shoulder length auburn hair. She wore a tight red sweater and black slacks.

Marjory spoke with a voice that belonged exclusively to the upper classes, and it soon became clear that she was not a lady to meddle with, only occasionally charming. Fred's offer of tenancy to Gwen could in no way have been a spur of the moment decision; he wouldn't have dared. It must have been planned with care, so arousing my suspicions. Marjory was telling me how they had two children of their own, both evacuated from the city for safety, when I realised that Fred and Gwen were no longer in the kitchen. They had moved somewhere else in the house. Somewhere private.

That evening, Marjory cooked a meal of steak followed by homemade apple pie. I didn't know how she had managed to get hold of this food, but everything was prepared to perfection. We sat in the dining room, drinking expensive red wine from Waterford crystal glasses, perched around an enormous mahogany table. Fred had the phonograph rigged up and was playing Debussy's *La Mer* at my request, which I had once seen performed with Eric. It should have been an enjoyable night, and probably was for Fred and Gwen. Marjory and I were excluded from their conversation, left to an increasingly awkward silence.

The distance to St. Peter's was now too great for cycling, and I had to resort to using the Underground. This was a real disappointment, a journey on the Metropolitan or Bakerloo Line no substitute for my previous cycle to work. On top of that, I missed my independence badly, hating to share a house with strangers. Fred had been quick to prove himself a little man in every respect, forever making little digs, attempting to prove himself my superior. It was getting on my nerves, and I could only put up with it in small doses. I never rushed to hurry from work. The only good thing when we moved to that house in Harrow was watching Gwen return to a semblance of her former self, all Garbo mannerisms and make-up. The problem was that it had nothing to do with me.

After one year of a so-called Phoney War, the first sporadic attacks on the city were being reported. It had been a long wait, but during September 1940 the Blitz on London began. My duties at the hospital alternated weekly between day and night shifts, and I watched the city transform quickly into a mess of fire and explosions.

German bombers arrived suddenly in huge numbers. An ominous drone in the sky fast became a heavy rain of incendiary devices. The air felt singed, choking the lungs, and London was sometimes lit up for miles. These attacks caused repeated damage to the railway tracks and walking became enforced.

Sometimes, it was easier to return to the hospital and sleep in the basement, although this was no safe haven. The walls were adorned with a spider web of hot water, waste, and steam pipes, and it was down to good luck alone that we received no direct hits.

It was a long hike back to Harrow, made unpleasant by the constant racket of explosions and tremors. If it should be quiet, anticipation filled any silence, making me equally tense and nervous. When I returned home, the four of us took to sleeping downstairs, barricaded into the front room with armchairs for added security. I don't know why this should have made a difference, offering no real protection from an attack, but it helped us all to sleep easier. I never forgot to carry Dot's bear.

It was a frightening time. We weren't yet used to the situation, and everybody began to collect stories that they wanted to relate, usually involving a close escape. Reg Marriott told how he had caught a taxi to meet with his wife in Soho. He had paid the fare, jumped out, and watched the very same cab blown into pieces as it rounded the corner. The driver's cap was thrown to his feet, which for reasons known only to Reg he had chosen to keep. He showed it to me; it was blue, wearing thin, with a shiny gold anchor embroidered into the peak.

I was walking to the hospital with him one night, along Whitechapel Road, when an air raid erupted about us. The streets were unlit, making it more difficult for enemy planes to locate their targets, and I found this to be a desperate measure. With all lights blacked out, I now even felt claustrophobic outside. Instinctively, we started to run.

Anti-aircraft guns shook the air, generating a warm wind. The ground shuddered beneath our feet, and I was aware of every jolt of my legs on the hard stone pavement. Shrapnel and slates began to rain from the sky, and I determined not to look up. My gaze fixed to the ground, I broke into a desperate sprint.

Mere seconds had passed when a cry sounded. A cry that stopped me dead. I turned to spot Reg had fallen outside The Grave Maurice, where he clutched his right leg in agony. I'd begun to go back, to help him, when another blast detonated from a bomb that landed nearby. I was blown clean off my feet and straight through a shop window, which fortunately had lost its glass on a previous raid. I looked up through the roof to see ragged bricks and cold blue stars, a far cry from the diamond sparkle of nights enjoyed with Eric Reynolds. A distant voice carried through the air. It was high-pitched, belonging to an old lady. 'Lavender. Lavender. Buy your lavender for luck.'

Strangers began to talk, to wish each other good fortune. The people of London stuck together in determined fashion, our job to stop the progress of Hitler. I would have expected the Blitz to push Gwen and me together, but this did not happen. It pulled us apart. When she drew the blackout blinds in our room, it left us circling each other like strangers or fish in a bowl. I watched, passive, while she grew ever closer to Fred, preferring to sit in his rooms than remain in my company. She knew that I would not follow, stubbornly determined to protect my precious privacy.

When attacks on the city intensified, thousands chose to shelter in the Underground stations at night, believing themselves to be safer below the ground. Huddled together like wraiths, or rows of lost souls, I had to step very carefully in order to avoid the jumble of bodies on my way to and from the hospital. Some people even managed to sleep sprawled lengthways down the stairs, and I grimaced at the thought of their discomfort in the morning. No arrangements had been provided by the authorities, and the smell of the unwashed was terrible. It could make me gag. They slept fitfully, resting on blankets and old newspapers, one arm or leg sometimes jerking out as I stumbled past them up the staircase. It was an unsettling sight, one I could never grow used to.

I could never escape from the sound of glass crumpling underfoot, the awful charred smell of the air. Buildings collapsed all about us, emptying their contents into streets where children played wild on the ruins. London eyes were weighed down by a haunted look of endless weariness, and I imagined ghosts wandering through the air, caught out by the sudden unfairness of death. These shoals of shadows darted in and out of the ruined buildings, unsure where they should go, for yesterday they had been alive. Anxiety and loss of sleep were definitely taking their toll. Work at the hospital continued to be as busy as ever, and rest was not an option.

I tried to understand what bound me to Gwen, and the war had a large part to do with it. In the carelessness of having no future, it was easier to remain together than actually separate, to avoid the hassle of splitting up. If I was going to die, like so many others, what did it matter if we remained together? I was not concerned about my future. It did not occur to me that each morning I was still alive and breathing, that the war would one day end.

All traces of romance had evaporated since the move to Harrow. Gwen became increasingly irritated at most aspects of my behaviour, and I could never seem to please her. She was no longer interested in sex, rotating the excuses of not in the mood, tiredness, her time, and I could not remember when we had last made love. Our conversation was strained and difficult, although she managed this well enough with Fred. I could no longer bring myself to listen to the songs we had once enjoyed. The music now seemed to mock me, jeering at my inability to sustain this relationship.

It was a definite relief to both of us when the conscription notice arrived. I would finally escape and get away. Gwen attributed her behaviour and lack of warmth to the stresses of war and sharing our accommodation, but I did not believe this. I remained suspicious of Fred, and it was obvious that Marjory had also noticed something. But as far as I was concerned, he was welcome to her.

The last time that I had seen Gwen was on the platform of a crowded Waterloo Station. Many men were being waved off to fight, and the noise was tremendous. White handkerchiefs waved in the air, and tears rolled down flushed, swollen faces. We tried to make our own farewell suitably reluctant and sincere. Gwen even kissed me, just the once.

'Look after yourself, Harold,' she said.

'You take care, Gwen. You'll be all right?'

'I'll be thinking of you.'

'Goodbye, then.'

'Goodbye.'

The word love was never mentioned. In truth, by the time I left England our relationship was long since finished. In reality, we had nothing left to say to each other.

CHAPTER FOURTEEN

I woke early, to a lilac morning. The sun shone into my eyes through the central of the three windows. I could see white clouds piled high in the sky; the distant sea was changed to violet. It was good to be on Malta, away from everything back home, and I knew that Nan wouldn't take long to arrive. She could show me Marsaxlokk and I hoped to make a good impression with her family. I might have been pumped full of medicine, but her love alone flowed in my veins.

Sitting upright, my insides sent out a warning flicker of pain. I still felt raw and bruised, a little weak, but I was determined to make it out of the villa. One of the other patients was resting, propped up against his pillow, and reading a book. The second man appeared to be asleep.

'All right, mate?' I called softly. 'What they got you in here for?'

He turned and nodded briefly, but said nothing. Nurse Vella must have been sitting directly outside the door, for I heard the immediate stomping of her feet across the tiles. She was a little cannonball of a woman, all dark, shiny, and round.

'Awake are we Fisher?' She approached my bed. 'And already disturbing the other patients. We can't be having that.'

To my relief, she smiled kindly. 'So how are you feeling today?'

'Much better, thanks. I slept great.'

'Good, good.' She rested one hand on the bed. 'It was a quiet night. Well I'd better get your temperature then, and have you taken your prescription?'

Breakfast consisted solely of toast and chlorinated tea. I tried again to start a conversation with my fellow inmates, but their eyes had turned inwards, away from both war and the world. They remained silent.

'You won't get a peep out of them,' Nurse Vella explained. 'That's why I put you by the door, as far away as I could. They're both recovering from burns, got them in Valletta. So are you going outside then? I haven't got all day to stop and chat.'

She helped me to the terrace, with a warning to be careful of the sun. 'It's the breeze you've got to watch out for. I don't want to be treating you for sunburn now!' And then she left me alone, at last, in blissful peace.

The wind curled noisily about the bay, and I surveyed the opposite headland. It was a perfect distance for swimming, if only I felt better. There was a man exercising on the beach directly in front of me, wearing a white vest and loose fitting black trousers. From where I sat, I could tell he was in excellent shape, a solid block of muscle. Press-ups, sit-ups, squats, and lunges; it was tiring just to watch him. I returned my attention to the bay.

I was able to watch the sea change from violet to green to a vivid iris blue as the day progressed. The fishing boats continued to bob tirelessly up and down. Each was painted in stripes of blue, yellow, green, red, and sometimes brown. Seabirds squawked about the harbour, ever hopeful and hungry for food; the sun rose and fell in the sky. All day, my thoughts were only of Nan.

On the following morning, I felt much improved. Nurse Vella had allowed me to dress, and I spotted the same man exercising on the beach. I decided to walk down and introduce myself, desperate to talk with somebody. My fellow patients remained mute and uncommunicative.

I stumbled down the track, towards the swirling blue and white sea. The man noticed and stopped his workout, bending to pick up a large white towel. He mopped rivers of sweat from his body, and I was able to see that he was tall, well built, with slicked thick black hair reminiscent of Eric Reynolds. The only real difference in appearance was that this man sported a moustache.

'Morning, how are you?' He spoke with a strong Cockney accent. 'Saw you arrive a couple of days ago.'

'Morning. I'm fine thanks, getting better. I'm glad to get out, it's like a morgue in there!'

'I'm sure,' he grinned, 'but not a bad spot this.' The little beach was sheltered by rocks on both sides, the shallow water pellucid green and reflecting the sun so brightly that it hurt my eyes. The wind from yesterday had nearly disappeared, its moan now reduced to a whisper.

'It's lovely,' I replied. 'I'm Harry Fisher, pleased to meet you.'

'Likewise.' He shook my hand with bone-crunching strength. 'So where you from then, Harry?'

'M'tarfa. I was stationed in the hospital up there, until I got ill. Be glad to get back. And you?'

'Sandy Goodacre, at your service mate!' He bowed and laughed, possessing a cackle that reminded me of Dicky Fuller. It made me like him immediately.

'I'm the senior NCO down here Harry, and the physical training instructor. Always enjoy my exercise in the morning, gets the day off to a good start. Do you do much yourself, mate? You look in reasonable shape.'

'I like to, when I can. But it's been too busy lately.' I turned towards the sea. 'I miss swimming more than anything. And walking. But I've always loved swimming, right from being a boy.'

'Me too, Harry. I've got a canoe down here, made it myself. We'll have to take it out when you're feeling up to it.'

'Sounds good, thanks Sandy.' Marsaxlokk appeared so peaceful and idyllic that it was hard to think of the war. 'So what's it been like down here, then? Seen much action?'

'Have we! Not half! It was bleeding awful, Harry. Only good thing was when a bomb landed in the harbour, stunned all the fish, it did. We had lovely fresh food for days, they all rose to the surface. And that reminds me, mate, I'm friends with one of the farmers down here, and he's always keen to barter.' We still received army rations of biscuits, bacon, jam, and bully beef. 'He'll give you the best grapes you've ever tasted for a few tins of food. Vegetables are good, too.' He patted his flat, firm stomach. 'Help you keep in shape!'

Sandy departed for work and left me alone on the beach. I looked back at the three villas, but everything was quiet up there. I wondered if the other houses also contained recovering patients.

The sea whispered in my ears, inviting, and I kicked off my shoes and socks - it still hurt to bend down. I paddled in the clear water, little fish darting near to my feet, and I continued to think about Nan. It was terrible to be away from her, a waste of precious time. I looked up into the sky and saw nothing but endless blue. It was all wind and air, with enemy attacks remaining thankfully scarce.

It was the fourth day when I was woken from my sleep. A hand shook me on the shoulder and I heard a frantic male voice.

'Come on Harry, get up. There's someone here to see you.'

Sandy stood beside the bed. He wore his usual clothes for exercise, a mischievous grin on his face.

'Who is it?' I croaked, my throat dry. My eyelids struggled to lift open.

'She's a real looker! Good on you, mate!' He slapped my shoulder hard with the palm of his hand. 'You never mentioned her!'

I jumped out of bed, becoming entangled in the sheet. My clothes were grabbed from a nearby chair and shoved on in record time; the usual khaki shirt and shorts. I tried to smooth down my hair, simultaneously rubbing my eyes in an attempt to wake up, while Sandy watched in obvious amusement. A broad smile creased his features, his head shaking slowly from side to side.

'Thanks, Sandy! I owe you one!' I rushed past him.

'Harold,' he called out, 'aren't you going to put on any shoes?'

She sat on the beach with her hands about both knees, toes curling to grasp into bare sand. Her face was turned to the sea. I had nearly reached her when I tripped, dislodging a large stone, and she twisted around at this disturbance.

'Hello, Harry, a horrible little woman wouldn't let me come inside. Your friend saw, and said he'd go and get you. He seemed nice.'

'Nan.'

She stood and smiled when I drew her to me. We were able to embrace, at last, and to kiss. My hands reached over each other on the small of her back, locking her against me.

'So are you feeling any better?' She tried to move, to look at me properly, but I wasn't letting go. 'Your strength is obviously coming back!' She laughed.

'I feel much better. Now. It's so good to see you, Nan.' We

kissed again. She wore a dark brown dress that I had not seen before. It was close fitting, cut just below knee length. 'You look great!' I buried my face in her hair. 'You smell great, too! In fact, you haven't changed at all. God, I've missed you!'

She placed one finger over my lips. 'So are you really feeling better, Harry?'

'Definitely. Much better.'

'And I'm here now.' She smiled. I continued to hold her close, one hand now resting over her bottom, the other stroking her back.

'So how are you, Nan? How's life at the old hospital?'

'It's a lot quieter. That's how I was able to get away.'

'Have you been to see your family?'

'No, I came straight here. The sea looks lovely.' She changed the subject, gazing over my shoulder. 'Are you allowed to swim yet? It seems like ages since we went.'

Nan held onto my arm when I released the grip on her back. We looked at the blue-green water caressing the beach. I remembered every second spent at our cove near Buskett Gardens, every second of our love.

'Not yet. I wish I could, but you go in. I'll watch.' The three villas appeared deserted. There was nobody else around.

Nan wriggled her shoulders, adjusting the straps of her dress that fell readily to the ground. She stepped free, her lithe tanned body clad only in white underclothes. Quickly, she walked into the shallows. The sun was already high in a deep blue sky. Little birds darted singing above my head, and I watched Nan disappear among the waves.

She possessed grace such that her body stroked the water, leaving it undisturbed. She moved rapidly, sometimes diving beneath the surface, as elusive as an apparition. When she came out from the sea, her auburn waterfall of hair dripped rainbows. A large white butterfly fluttered behind her head, following her every move. Tiny yellow flowers floated by her feet, and I stood frozen still. Transfixed.

'Nan', I spoke softly, removing my shirt and handing it to her for use as a towel. 'You're beautiful.' She smiled and I placed a finger onto her birthmark, tracing the outline. 'You're perfect.'

'Shut up, Harry! You're making me embarrassed.'

'But I mean it. You are.'

We sat huddled on rocks to the right of the beach, and I placed my arm about her shoulders, kissing the moist nape of her neck. I always loved the salt taste of her skin after she'd been swimming.

'So are you going to show me Marsaxlokk, then?'

'Not today, Harry. We'll wait until you're better, and I've got some more time. But there's one thing I did want to show you - look!' She pointed to the nearest of the painted fishing boats. 'See that at the front, that mark?'

'What is it Nan?'

'It's an eye, like they have in Egypt, to ward off evil spirits. I think it's a good thing, yes?'

'Maybe we should paint one on each other, Nan?'

'I already have! That's why I wanted to show you. It's right in the middle of your back.' I craned my neck, attempting to look, but Nan slapped me on the arm. 'It's invisible, silly! I did it with my finger, after we'd first met.'

She managed to stay with me until noon, when her ride to M'tarfa had been arranged. It was horrible to let her go, but she promised to return soon. When I was with Nan, I felt my strength returning quickly. Outside, by the sea, I felt like my normal self again. It was only inside the villa with my silent companions that I felt like an invalid.

Sandy Goodacre returned in the afternoon, and found me sitting on the rocks.

'Blimey, Harry, you want to be careful. You're looking a bit pink. You'll burn away to nothing if you stay out here.'

'Sorry, mate, I was miles away.' I jumped at his approach. As usual, I had been thinking about Nan.

'C'mon, we'll find you some shade.' Sandy waited for me to climb to my feet. 'I'll show you that canoe.'

He skirted a route to the left of the beach, where we scrambled over rocks and rounded a corner, out of sight of the villas. Another cove glistened in front of us, even more sheltered than the previous one. Here, the calm water resembled cut glass, the faintest shade of blue, and the surface so smooth that I believed I could walk upon it. A small wooden hut was located near to where we stood, positioned beneath tall silver olive trees. Sandy produced a key from his pocket, brandishing this with pride.

'Nice little set-up I've got here, eh? Thought you'd like to see it.' He unlocked the hut, which seemed an unnecessary precaution. It was so well hidden. 'After you, mate.'

Sandy stepped aside and I entered the cabin. Inside, a small bed had been fashioned from old wooden crates that were covered with a thin mattress. The canoe lay on the floor, carved crudely out of an old tree trunk. It was designed to seat two people.

'Thought you could use this place next time your lady comes to visit. I'll let you keep the key.'

'Thanks Sandy. It's fantastic.'

'I know! I've used it once or twice myself. And it gets even better.' He laughed, that familiar cackle, as he rolled the canoe onto its side. Underneath, lay several cool bottles of Blue Label beer and a bottle opener.

'Your health, mate! Cheers!'

'Cheers!'

We were able to reminisce about London. Sandy actually came from the East End, where he shared a house with his mother. He knew St. Peter's Hospital well. I told him how I liked the area, but was never keen on Cable Street.

'No, no mate. A nasty business that. And you want to watch out for Brick Lane, too. A bunch of thieves down there.'

I told him about Eric Reynolds; he seemed flattered at this comparison, and how we used to go drinking along the Whitechapel Road.

'Used to go there sometimes myself, Harry,' he replied. 'But not much mind.'

'Not good for keeping in shape, right?'

'That's right, Harry!' He grinned, delighted. 'That's right!'

We took the canoe out on the following afternoon, sneaking from the villa like naughty schoolboys. We rowed for hours, capsizing often, and only the onset of darkness put a stop to our fun. I was feeling better by the day, but Nurse Vella still gave me a blasting when I returned to bed. It was too early for 'pranks like that' in her opinion, but I didn't care. She could not be right about everything. That night, my sleep came sweetly and easy.

An air raid took place in the morning, the first one since arrival in Marsaxlokk. Even the mighty Nurse Vella must have realised that I was recovering when she discovered me dragging the mattresses from the floor to cover and protect my fellow patients. I chose to watch this spectacle outside, on the terrace, and saw two German planes pass overhead in the direction of Valletta. No bombs were dropped near us.

It was not long after that these same planes were spotted in hasty retreat, pursued by two of our Spitfires. It was then that I knew I was definitely ready to return to F Block. I wanted to be back at work, pulling my weight again, playing my part in the war.

The afternoon was spent in frustration, prowling around the villa with nothing able to occupy me. Sandy was nowhere to be seen. I couldn't read or write a letter - it was far too inactive a task. I wanted to be doing something more useful, something practical. It was incredibly irritating to be kept away from the heart of things, and I was becoming more and more impatient. I did not even notice Nan's arrival.

'Hello Harry.' She approached from behind, wrapping arms about my stomach, leaning her head against my back.

'Nan. I wasn't expecting you.' It was the middle of the afternoon. 'How did you get here now?'

I turned around, taking her hands in my own. She smiled but quickly looked away, gazing out towards the bay.

'I had the day free.' She hesitated. 'I've been to see my family.'

'But Nan,' I exploded, all impatience and frustrations boiled over, 'I thought you were going to take me! I thought I was going to meet them at last. You knew that. Why didn't you come and get me?' My voice was ugly and strange with rage.

'I was going to, but then...'

'It's like you're embarrassed about me,' I cut in. 'Or ashamed. What's the point in any of this if that's what you really think?'

'I don't think that, Harry. It's not that simple.'

'What is it then?' I continued to shout.

'Because,' she spoke slowly, almost inaudible, 'I'm a Catholic.'

'So what? I thought we loved each other.'

'It would matter to them, Harry.' She looked into my eyes, pleading for understanding.

'Do they even know about me?' Realisation struck like an unexpected fist. Nan appeared crestfallen.

'No,' she whispered.

I stormed away, without once glancing backwards, heading straight for my room. It seemed inconceivable that she had not even mentioned me, anger having stolen all reasoning. My pride was in tatters. Nan meant everything. She was my world; if I was anything to her, I couldn't understand how she would remain silent and keep our relationship a secret.

Crashing into the room, I sat heavily on the bed. For once, I was glad that my companions would not speak. Nan was outside, somewhere, and I was furious. With her, the war, and myself. War was mainly an emotion, I realised this, unknown until experienced, and I did not like what it was doing to me.

Nan was outside, the woman who I loved. Nan was outside. Surely that was the only thing that mattered. She had come to see me. Things were different here; even Dicky had told me that, right at the beginning. I could not hope to understand everything. But Nan was outside, and I knew that I loved her. Nan was outside.

I stood up to retrace my steps. She waited by the door, prohibited to enter the villa. Her eyes were red and tears ran freely down both cheeks.

'I'm sorry, Nan.' I pulled her against me, and felt her arms reach tight about my back. 'I'm so sorry. I'm just sick of all this, and being away from you.'

'I know. I know,' she murmured, her voice broken with emotion. 'Me too. I'm sorry, I should have told them about you.'

'That's okay. Another time. Come on, let's get away from here.' I took her hand. She wore a pale grey skirt and brown top, a straw hat clutched tightly over her chest. Nan managed a smile and I kissed the tip of her nose.

'There's something I've got to show you.'

I took her to Sandy's hideout, a short walk from the villa. When we stood in front of the hut, I made her close her eyes while I unlocked the door.

'Your room, madam! Nan, you can look now.'

'Oh Harry, it's wonderful!' Her laughter filled the air.

'Not quite the Ritz, but at least we've got some privacy. Come on, let's take the canoe out. I want to go swimming with you.'

We rowed together, Nan sitting in front, each daring the other in an attempt to stand upright. Sandy's canoe invariably rolled over, throwing us quickly into the water. My shorts refused to stay up; I had lost weight after all, causing Nan considerable merriment. Her laughter arrived in joyous explosions.

At the frayed edge of sunset, we made love in the saltwater. It felt like coming home. We sat on the beach while darkness drenched into the day, discussing the useless pain of war and, more important, how lucky we were to have found each other. Nothing could tear us apart. Nothing could or would go wrong. I had never seen so many stars pierce through the indigo sky.

CHAPTER FIFTEEN

The time allowed for convalescence sped past, and after one week I was delighted to report back to Major Merryweather at the hospital. The driver had allowed me to sit with him in the cab on the return journey to M'tarfa, and I had experienced a real sense of exhilaration to spot Mdina rising in the distance. This had quickened into jubilation as we twisted through Rabat, plunging down into the valley that led up to the hospital. The Major waited in his office. To my amazement, I realised that I had even begun to miss the smell of disinfectant.

'How are you doing, Harold? You've got some colour again, I'm glad to see.' The Major walked forward to greet me with his usual handshake.

'I'm much better, thank you.' It was true. I hadn't felt this good for months. My body raced with rediscovered health. I felt strong again.

'So are you ready to return to us?'

'Definitely, yes!'

'Well, we'd better have a look at you then.'

He led me into the nearest ward, where some of the beds remained empty. I kept my fingers crossed during this examination, reaching instinctively for Dot's bear in my shirt pocket. Through the window behind his head, I could see the twin belfries of the cathedral in Mdina, imagining them to represent Nan and me. The towering ancient stone, unbroken through long years, seemed to epitomise our love. It was built to last, and very beautiful.

The Major seemed to be happy with this inspection, murmuring words of approval more to himself than for my benefit. When he palpated above my liver, it hardly hurt at all. He stood abruptly, nodding his head.

'Right then Harold, I've some bad news for you.' My heart sank. 'I think you're big enough, ugly enough, and strong enough for the treatment to be repeated. I'm sure you were expecting that.'

'No. I wasn't.' In my illness I had forgotten that this would be necessary. The mere thought of a sigmoidoscope, and that bastard RMO, was enough to make me want to turn and run naked all the way to Marsaxlokk.

'We'll have you back properly after that.' He patted my shoulder, removing his spectacles. 'Don't worry, Harold, it's nowhere near as bad the second time.'

He was telling me the truth. The treatment was carried out immediately, and I did not have to wait long before I was deemed fit enough to resume control of F Block. It was strange to sleep in my bed in the barracks again, dark and uncomfortable after the room in the villa, but it was with delight that I walked down St. David's Road to work. Each of the little houses struck me as impossibly charming, thankfully unscathed in my absence. Butterflies whirled in the warm air, a strip of blue sea always visible on the horizon.

Entering through the gates to the hospital, the main building displayed an acne of gunshot damage although it was generally intact. I passed the chapel quickly, eager to resume my duties, but stopped to touch the sign outside the building. F Block; I had returned and this felt wonderful. I took one deep breath and opened the door with a flourish.

Sister Merciecp was sitting at the desk. She looked up and a huge smile graced her features. I felt my own face crease and tighten in reply.

'Olivia.'

'Hello Harold!' We met in the centre of the ward, hugging briefly. 'We'd been told you were coming.'

'And it's great to be back, I can tell you.'

'It's good to have you back. We've been looking after the place for you.' She continued to smile. 'So how are you feeling?'

'Fine. Fine.' I studied the ward, now preoccupied. We had few empty beds, but the room seemed unnaturally quiet. The atmosphere was calm, and two nurses walked along the central aisle checking on each of the patients. They turned towards me, waving in recognition. I held up one hand in greeting. 'So has there been much change, Olivia? Have we the same staff?'

'It's been better, Harold. Much better. We're back to the usual admissions. We haven't needed the iron lung, and yes, we've kept the same nurses.' That was why the ward was so quiet. I missed the mechanical cough and wheeze of the Nuffield Drinker, the squeak of the bellows, but only for one second. It meant that we had no new cases of polio to look after. 'Someone's been looking after us, Harold. We could have done much worse.'

'That's good news, Olivia. And thank you.' I touched her elbow. 'Well, I'd better get started then!'

It was with continued joy and delight that I set enthusiastically about this ward inspection. Standards remained high, and I was pleased to note the thick layer of grease smeared over bed legs, the water-filled tins on the ground, the excellent degree of cleanliness. It was no mean feat after the shortages of water and soap. The building had also been repaired, with doors and windows patched up, the insect control mesh again functional.

All patients appeared to be comfortable, and there were several whom I recognised. A further change was evident, creeping into the eyes of these men, which I noticed immediately. Their skin was now old, shrunken and yellow, yet their eyes had acquired a childlike wonder at the world. Everything appeared to them as fresh and new.

I remembered the pain and despair of polio, the agony of strong, young men grown helpless. Now, I watched the return of hope mixed with disbelief at actually getting better. These men had a future again, something previously doubted, and they stared in unblinkered astonishment through the windows of the building.

We had no patients upstairs, my own bed empty, but I still cursed the RMO for good measure. I hoped that one day he would be admitted, that he might need use of a sigmoidoscope, and then I could get my own back. I glanced down at my hands, noticing that they were covered with the usual limestone dust. It was also on my shirt and trousers. I must have leaned against the wall and I cursed this too, although I didn't really mind. With the inspection completed, even the paperwork brought me pleasure.

Restored to M'tarfa, it was far easier to arrange meetings with Nan. Her own duties on Surgical had grown much lighter, and we were able to return to Buskett Gardens. This we did often. The barracks remained crowded but here we were able to love until morning, resting on her bamboo mat, under a night sky studded with stars. On the occasions I slept alone, without Nan to hold, I didn't know what to do with my hands.

I was able to visit Valletta for the first time in months. Hitching a lift to the top end of Kingsway, the Opera House remained in ruins. That burned, charred smell in the air was thankfully absent. The population of the city went about their daily business, and I was able to admire their fortitude and determination. It had been much the same in London. Several shops had re-opened and there was considerable evidence of a clean-up operation in progress. Streets that had previously been obstructed were now accessible, cleared of most rubble. I heard music playing inside apartments, the sound of laughter, and decided to visit Fort St. Elmo. My intention was to enjoy the view across the harbour towards Sliema.

Approaching the Services Club, in the shade of one of the old palaces, a shout disturbed my walk. The voice was familiar, one that I'd long hoped to hear in the city.

'Harry Fisher! Blimey, mate, can't get rid of you then!'

This was followed with a raucous cackle and I spun around, delighted.

'Dicky! I haven't seen you for ages. I heard about the Regent Cinema and I was getting worried.'

'The Regent, a bad business that.' For once, he looked serious, but this was only in passing. 'So are you going to buy me a drink then?'

'Too right, I am.'

I clapped my arm about his shoulders and we started across the square to reach the club. Dicky looked thinner, older, his face drawn tight with the memory of hunger. But most people looked like this; it was nothing unusual. His green eyes still sparkled, along with his wit.

'So how's the woman, then? Keeping all right, Harry?' We stopped to allow a karozzin trundle slowly past, its wheels clacking loudly over the damaged stone of the road. Both our heads turned to watch the horse drop a giant stream of manure across our path. Dicky looked at me and winked.

'Reminds me of a joke that, Harry.' He roared with laughter as we entered the Union Jack. 'Can't beat a good joke, eh Harry?'

We ordered two bottles of Blue Label, toasting each other's good health. Dicky told me how he'd remained in Valletta, manning one of the gunposts. The casualties had been heavy, and he'd hated not being able to retaliate while siege restrictions affected ammunition supply. Many of his company were now dead.

We drank quickly. I looked about the room; despite it being early afternoon, the bar was already filled with men. An excited chatter filled the air, free of recent gloom, and this proved to be infectious. We ordered another two beers, this time toasting the women, although I was only thinking of one.

'But you should have seen *Ohio*, Harry' Dicky continued. 'What a sight! She was nearly going under, but she saved our bacon. Been abandoned twice, a big hole in her side, she was carried into the harbour.'

'And the Gozo farmers,' I was quick to point out. 'They helped, too.'

'For food, yes, but *Ohio* brought ammunition. Anyway, did you hear who's playing tonight?'

'Who?' The Entertainment's National Service Association had started visits to the island, attempting to raise morale. It was an organisation of actors and singers that had quickly acquired a nickname amongst the men. I wouldn't have been surprised if Dicky himself had made this up.

'Every Night Something Awful, eh Harry?' He laughed with glee. 'But not tonight. They've got George Formby on at Kala Frana. Do you fancy coming, I've got a ride all sorted?'

'Why not? Sounds good.'

It was a Maltese pal of Dicky's who drove us to the south of the island, near the airstrip at Hal Far, in plenty of time for the show. He dropped us off at a bay that looked surprisingly familiar. I stared at the headland in the distance, across the clear powder blue water. A small town and harbour, a jumble of houses, were clearly visible.

'Know where that is, Harry?' Dicky joined me after his friend had departed in a cloud of swirling dust. 'Delimara Point. A good spot for a swim, that.'

I felt glad to have accepted his offer, for I was once again returned near to Nan's home. This occasion was infinitely preferable to being sent on sick leave. I looked at the dots of colour bobbing and weaving on the surface, the little fishing boats, wondering which one belonged to her father. I still waited to meet with the man.

'Come on, mate, let's go. Have to get us some decent seats.'

George Formby kept us laughing throughout a long night, singing and joking in a smoky room within the barracks, until his voice packed up completely. Sitting next to Dicky and his contagious cackle, my insides felt bruised from too much laughter. Many of the men seemed to be chuckling as much at Dicky's good humour as the efforts of George Formby, and it was a pleasure to be his companion. My prayer for his safety had most definitely been answered.

Joyce Grenfell was my favourite visitor, not long after this. She attended unit dances for both officers and the men in M'tarfa, bringing her charm and considerable talent to the bedside of those patients unable to attend the performances. I felt privileged to act as her guide around F Block, watching closely as she brought laughter to the ward. This was the toughest audience of all, but she reached deeply into the men, pulling them up and out of their sickness. Her songs and comic monologues helped to forget the horrors experienced, to think back, and hopefully forwards, to better times.

The Italian Navy surrendered in Malta in September 1943, this story spreading quicker than any wind or the gossip of old ladies. For a long time, it had seemed they would surely be arriving as our conquerors. It was fantastic news to hear.

Work kept me in M'tarfa, but a few of us collected on the hospital roof in the hope of observing something. It was a glorious day, the heat becoming more bearable after the ferocity of summer, and it did not matter that we could not really see anything. Most of the action took place in Valletta, but some of their fleet anchored in St. Paul's Bay, a distant blur on our horizon. There was no mistaking the sweep of excitement across the island, and I had Nan to share this with me.

During the siege, there had been occasional reports of how the Maltese had evicted Brits from their shelters, complaining they were only under attack due to our presence. Now, hospitality was universally tremendous. Everybody believed that the island had achieved something remarkable, surviving the siege, polio, and countless attacks. Wining, dining, and dancing, became a nightly occurrence, with one of the biggest events hosted at the hospital.

All day, we took turns preparing the large dining hall for evening. Tables and chairs were cleared from the centre of the floor, a makeshift stage constructed at one end of the room. Coloured paper strips were stuck onto the walls, to provide a faint illusion of glamour. The hours passed so slowly, I couldn't wait for the dance to arrive. My uniform was washed and ironed with unusual care and attention.

The sun hung low in the sky, casting a deep orange glow across M'tarfa, when I met Nan outside her quarters. It was still warm and the birds were out in force, singing noisily. I stood behind an olive tree, humming *Red Sails*, until I heard her door open and close, the sound of shoes clicking over the stone.

Nan appeared wearing a lily-white dress, her hair tied back elaborately, two corkscrews of fringe hanging on either side of her face. She wore heels, the first time I had seen this, her legs made even more lovely. She smiled, and tiny diamond earrings glittered and sparkled with sunlight. Fragile, delicate straps of the dress covered both shoulders, revealing her dusky olive skin.

'Wow. You look amazing!' I walked forwards, her hands reaching out for me. 'I'm afraid to touch you, in case I mess anything up.'

'Don't be silly,' she squeezed my fingers. 'You'd better kiss me right now, or you'll be in big trouble Mr Fisher.'

Our lips met. She tasted of toothpaste and something sweet. I smelled her hair, the usual musk, and felt for her bottom through the thin silk of the dress. 'Really Nan, you look wonderful.'

'Thanks Harry, you look nice too.'

I felt woefully underdressed to accompany her. If Eric had been there, he would surely have located a dinner jacket from somewhere, and for once his partner would have been no match for my own. I offered Nan my arm and we idled slowly along St. David's Road. Sporadic bursts of music were already audible from the hospital. The band was tuning up.

'Italy down, we're going to win then Nan, just like you said.' I still couldn't quite believe it, the siege too fresh in my memory.

'I know, Harry, but let's not talk about war tonight. Let's just enjoy ourselves.'

Other couples walked towards the hospital, and cars were beginning to arrive from all directions. I glanced to my left, towards Mdina, admiring the way it climbed majestically above the patchwork of fields. Beyond this lay Valletta and the Mediterranean sea. I was affected with a deep love of the island that had brought me such happiness, such a woman, and turned to kiss Nan extravagantly on the cheek.

'What was that for?'

'No reason. Just felt like it.' I squeezed her arm. 'This is the first time I've been able to take you out properly, isn't it? I can't wait to show you off.'

'I've been happy all the time, Harry. You can't beat Buskett Gardens, I like it when we're alone.'

'I know, but tonight we can dance. I should let you know that I'm a very good dancer.'

'Is that true?' She looked at me, enquiring. 'You've never told me that before.'

'Well, no. But watch me fly tonight!'

We reached the gates to the hospital at the exact same time as an army van screeched up the dirt track from Mdina. It came straight at us before braking at the very last minute, skidding, shooting dust against my legs. I jumped in front of Nan, to protect her from this dirt. The van door popped open, and out jumped Dicky Fuller accompanied with two heavily made-up beauties.

'All right, Harry!' He grinned. Dicky looked immaculate in evening wear, bending low to adjust the crease of his trousers. His black shoes appeared as polished as marble.

'Dicky! How did you get here? And where did you get that suit? It's good to see you.'

'You know me Harry' he chuckled. 'Never like to miss a dance. See you inside, eh?' He took a lady on each arm and positively jogged up the path to the hospital. I looked at Nan and grinned.

'He's unbelievable, isn't he?'

'He brought us together, so yes.' She kissed me on the lips. 'So are we going inside?'

The dining hall and guests were unrecognisable, all officers wearing dinner jackets and their ladies suitably glamorous. Lights were dimmed and the coloured paper prettied the walls. One table had been converted into a bar, where people now queued for drinks. I began to edge towards this when the band suddenly stopped their tuning and struck up the first song, scattering the audience about the room.

'Come on, Nan' I grabbed her to me. 'Let's try a waltz.'

Nan danced so freely, easily; it was as if the music came from inside her. She smiled when I held her close, growing ever more ambitious, executing ostentatious spin turns to the fine music. One song blended into another, and still we danced. Dicky appeared briefly, 'Floor's not bad eh?' he muttered and was gone. I felt that we would surely fly out of the window, up into the deep blue of the sky, to meet with the milky white stars. The room became a beautiful blur, and I imagined the Royal Albert Hall replacing the hospital dining room about us.

'I wouldn't have missed this for the world Harry,' Nan whispered into my ear, kissing the side of my face.

'No way, not for anything!'

We shone our love about the room for all to see, like the beam from a lighthouse, dancing foxtrots, waltzes, and my favourite, the quickstep.

To our amazement, we were awarded the prize of Best Couple, leading the hall in a special waltz. I could have been in heaven, I felt so ridiculously happy.

'There's something I've got to tell you, Nan.' I was getting out of breath.

'Can't it wait?' she sighed with mock annoyance.

'I love you!'

She held me closer. Dicky was waving and whistling from the side of the room, a girl still hanging on each arm. Life didn't get any better than this, and I was more than disappointed when the dance was brought to a close. The night was too young, too perfect, to relinquish.

'Let's go to the cove Nan.'

'I was going to say that!' She spoke with obvious excitement. We always seemed to be in tune with each other. 'But I'm not really dressed for walking. Shall we go and get changed first?'

'No need, I've got a better idea. I'll drive!'

The Major had allowed me this privilege before, of borrowing his Austin Utility van. It was parked nearby and I had hardly touched any alcohol, too busy with the dancing. We reached the vehicle quickly. It was unlocked as usual, keys dangling ready in the ignition.

The van had a single front bench seat that I brushed clean with one hand. Dust got everywhere on the island, and I didn't want to be responsible for ruining Nan's dress. It was stunning, and elegant. I'd never seen her look better.

'Your carriage, Madam.' I bowed, my head dipping low to the ground.

'Why thank you, Mr. Fisher.' She giggled and curtsied. I opened her door and we sat huddled together.

'Right then,' I turned to face her, our lips so close that I couldn't help but kiss her. 'If we're Best Couple, then that's how we're going to drive. All right?' I bent forwards to kiss her again, taking my time, wrapping my arm about her shoulders. 'I'll drive, but when it's time to change gears I'll shout 'now'. That's your job.'

'Yes sir!' This time, Nan kissed me. 'Ready, sir.'

The engine coughed hard and spluttered into life. I shouted, and Nan rammed home the gear-stick. We were off, laughing like maniacs, and I steered towards Mdina.

I nearly hit a rabbit as we sped out of Rabat, braking hard to avoid it, but we passed no other cars. The only scare was when we neared the Verdala Palace and I turned to kiss Nan, taking my eyes away from the road. 'Harry' she screamed, 'Watch out!' We narrowly avoided the iron gates, but she managed to twist the steering wheel just in time. I kissed her anyway, and soon we had reached the cliff tops. After a rapid descent, the cove was thankfully deserted.

There was no wind to disturb the silence. Nan had discarded her shoes by the side of the van and now walked with naked feet embracing the cool, pale sand. She told me I had looked svelte in the dance, tall and graceful, and it became my favourite word. The sea brushed lips gently over the beach.

We stopped walking. Nan's bare shoulders appeared exquisite in the moonlight. Stars shone in her hair and dark eyes. She took hold of my face between both hands, pulling downwards, to kiss me long and slow. And then she began to dance, the moon as her spotlight, and all I could make out was the dress shimmering so beautiful alone, floating ghost-like above the sand. The night itself seemed to pause and weigh anchor. My heart beat as slow as deep water.

Suddenly, Nan became still. Time slowed while the dress fell to the ground. I was so overcome with beauty and desire that it made my breath stop. I watched a shadow disappear into the hushed, black sea.

It did not take long to discard my own clothes and join her. Making love, I experienced complete peace and contentment. We returned to the van barefoot, hand in hand, and my whole body was soaring. Strange, beautiful music filled my head, and once again Nan held my face while kissing me. She broke off, whispering into the night, 'I can feel you are free, Harry. I love you.'

For the second time, I believed our love to be blessed.

Chapter Sixteen

I wanted to be with Nan all of the time. If I wasn't with her, I was thinking about her. I wanted to relate everything that I had done in her absence, and to hear every detail concerning what had happened to her. We had been together for over three years, with no sign at all of love waning. It would be there forever, like the sea, of this I felt convinced.

It was in the summer of 1944 that the first of our dreams came true, and we managed to obtain the same two weeks leave period. There was only one thing to do with our time, and that was to visit Gozo. It was finally going to happen.

I had arranged a lift to take us to the ferry landing at Cirkewwa, on the north of the island, and Nan thought that I must have planned it when a grinning Dicky Fuller raced up to the hospital entrance. I was amazed. I hadn't seen him for months.

'All right Harry! Nan!' He jumped out of a dusty, grey van, a huge dent crumpling the front bumper. 'Don't say I never do anything for you, eh? May I take your bags?'

These last words were spoken in a posh accent, Dicky standing to attention before bursting into his usual laughter. Our canvas rucksacks were thrown without ceremony into the boot of the van. 'Well come on then, get in! Haven't got all day, like some people!' He had regained his lost weight and looked to be in excellent health. It was great to see him, a perfect start to our trip.

'Dicky Fuller! How the hell did you manage to pull this one off?' We all sat together on the front seat.

'Friends in the right places, Harry,' he winked, tapping the side of his nose. 'And about that dance, when did you ever get so good? Going to Gozo, eh? Where are you staying?'

'The Duke of Edinburgh.'

'Only the best for Nan, eh? You were never so generous back home!' He roared with laughter, the van swerving dangerously to the side of the road. 'I told you, didn't I, that you'd like each other? Didn't know how much though, blimey!' He punched my arm, still grinning.

'So how's it been in Valletta, Dicky?'

We drove along narrow, twisting roads at treacherous speed. The sun dazzled my eyes. Nan remained silent, holding my hand, while our friend chatted happily, not waiting for any reply.

'Well they're not rebuilding yet, but the clean-up's coming on. It's a lot safer now, getting busy again. Was a lot quieter for a while, but the curfew's been relaxed. Just as well, a man's got to have a drink, eh? Bars are the only ones who've done all right in this business, and some of the women,' he nudged my side. 'Be sorry to leave the old place. Gets under your skin.'

In little time, the road came to a dead end where it met with the sea, and Dicky was depositing us on a bare patch of ground. A crude stone wall comprised the quay where our fellow passengers stood waiting; two round priests, apparently untouched by any siege, a farmer clad in faded overalls, and one black goat with a mischievous glint in its eyes.

'Thanks, Dicky. See you when we get back.'

He stuck his head through the open window of the van. 'You two have fun. Don't know which boat it is today, but it won't be long coming. Young love, eh? Ain't it grand!'

He smiled, revving the engine noisily, before skidding away and spraying me with dust in the process. I heard his laughter ringing in the hot air long after the vehicle had disappeared. Nan climbed onto the stone harbour wall, waiting for me to join her.

'Look, Harry. That's Gozo over there!' She pointed straight ahead as I cuddled her against me, where a teasing glimpse of green countryside and church spires flickered in the distance. The wind whipped her hair across my face, into my mouth and eyes. 'We're on our way at last. I told you we'd get there, didn't I?'

A small boat inched slowly towards the quay, one of the local fishing vessels. The sail was up and I could see that the captain wore dark shorts and a white shirt with rolled-up sleeves. Nobody else was onboard.

'Do you think that's it?' I asked Nan.

'I don't know. I hope so. The one I went on before, the *Royal Lady*, was terrible. It made me feel so sick. We all called it the rolling lady!'

'She was sunk,' one of the priests interrupted, speaking with a flawless English accent. 'Split into two at Mgarr. It's always these boats now. Are you long on Gozo?' A beatific smile illuminated his well-fed features.

'Two weeks, Father,' Nan answered.

'Well I am sure you will both enjoy it. And will you be visiting Ta Pinu?'

'Of course.' Nan played with the gold chain about her neck.

We embarked quickly, the goat leaping happily onto the deck, and the captain collected a fare of one shilling each. Nan and I sat at the back while the rest of the passengers lay down to nap, and soon we were on our way to the island. The sea under siege had sometimes taken on the hue of gunmetal, but now appeared a perfect aquamarine. I trailed one hand in

NIGHT SKY DREAMING

the cool water, holding onto Nan with the other.

The crossing took one hour, our boat sliding smoothly across the four miles that separated Gozo from Malta. We passed several other fishing vessels, the Gozitans onboard waving happily. A convoy of seabirds flew in the air behind us, hoping in vain for scraps of food.

'That's Comino, over there.' Nan tugged on my arm. 'Where they have the isolation hospital.'

I looked up to see a small, barren island, a single tower visible near the coast that we approached. An even smaller island was situated next to this, separated by rocks resembling the stepping-stones of a giant. The water between these islands was the most intense, startling blue.

'Wow, Nan! Look at the sea over there.'

'I know,' she followed my gaze. 'That's the Blue Lagoon. The swimming is wonderful there - we'll have to go.'

A skyline of distant villages, domed churches, and green fields, heralded the arrival of Gozo. A wash of quiet spilled into the harbour, and I liked it straight away. The port of Mgarr was compact and pretty, safely enclosed between low, rocky cliffs. Caves were visible, providing extra shelter for the many brightly painted fishing boats that bobbed gently at rest. A little beach nestled at the edge of the waterfront, and, to our left, a large fort stood at the highest point, commanding the channel between the islands.

We were able to hire a karozzin for the remaining part of our journey. I had booked us into The Duke of Edinburgh in Victoria, supposedly the best hotel on Gozo. Our driver flicked the reins, and with a jolt the carriage began to move. I felt sorry for the old horse, having to drag the three of us up a steep hill and away from the harbour.

A ride of half an hour confirmed the beauty of our

surroundings. The Gozitans who we passed walking along the road seemed uniformly friendly, shouting out greetings. Those working in the fields stopped what they were doing in order to wave at us. The pace of life appeared slow and unhurried, the countryside open and lovely. Even the light appeared different, possessing a clean, unusual clarity. I was short-sighted, but here this did not seem to affect me.

I had enjoyed my time on Malta, particularly the rush, bustle, and noise of the place. It had impressed me much as London first had in the Thirties, only more so. In no way, however, had it prepared me for the splendid tranquil beauty of Gozo. The karozzin trundled slowly into Victoria, large stone houses now lining both sides of the road.

'This is Racecourse Street, Harry.' Nan sounded excited. 'If we're lucky, we'll get to see them racing horses and buggies along here. Look over there!'

We had a good view of the city huddled like a child at the knees of the Citadel, a mighty fortress that rose vertical from a central position. Tiny dots identified people walking along the high battlements.

'I'll take you up there. The view from the top is very special, you can see the whole island. And it's great for sunsets.'

The karozzin jerked to a stop. Our driver jumped down and opened Nan's door.

'The Duke of Edinburgh. We are here,' he announced.

The hotel appeared a modest two-storey building from the outside, constructed of a sand-coloured stone. Colonnades of short pillars lined the rooftop, looking like a row of skittles waiting to be bowled over. Some of the rooms had balconies overlooking the street, the green shuttered windows all closed.

'Hello.' A man waved down from the roof. 'I'll be with you in one moment.'

He must have run all the way, for after we had paid the driver and gathered our bags he stood smiling at the hotel entrance.

'Welcome to the Duke of Edinburgh, sir, madam.' He bowed modestly. 'Mr. Fisher, I presume? I am Noel, and will show you to your room.'

'Call me Harry, we're going to be here for awhile. And this is Nan.'

'I'm sorry, sir, I'm not allowed to do that.'

He wouldn't let me carry our bags, either. Noel was a slim man, about forty years of age. He stood a similar six feet to myself, with wavy brown hair and a smart moustache. He wore a loose fitting white shirt with black trousers, his eyes shining with alertness and gentle good humour. 'Now if you will follow me.'

He led the way up broad, shallow stone steps, along a cool corridor, to the rear of the building. 'I wish you could have visited before the war, sir. The houses in front of us are new, and we used to have wonderful views across the island. This is your room.'

The bags were deposited carefully on the ground, a key was produced, and the door unlocked. 'I hope that you will be very happy here. If there is anything I can do, please let me know.' Another bow, and Noel departed. I pushed the door open and followed Nan inside.

She stood smiling in the centre of the room. A large iron bed occupied much of the space, covered with immaculate white sheets, white drapes hanging on either side. The walls were also a spotless white, the floor pale marble, and opposite the bed stood a large dressing table of dark wood.

The window was positioned at the end of the room, through which a radiant red bougainvillaea waved a hand. Our room overlooked gardens filled with pink and white oleander trees, wild jasmine, and trailing vines swaying like snakes in the breeze.

'Come here, you.' Nan spoke quietly, drawing me into a kiss. 'Welcome to Gozo.'

Clothes were removed and she pushed me backwards, onto the bed. She climbed on top of me, lowering herself slowly, before bending forwards. Her hair fell over my face, I loved that, and I was able to take her breasts into my mouth. She never once took her eyes from my face, looking at me all through our lovemaking.

It was late in the afternoon when we eventually left the hotel. Nan continued to chat happily as I dragged her towards the Citadel.

'You'll like it here, Harry, I'm sure. The people speak differently to Malta - see if you can notice. Even here in Victoria, there are two accents. They're quieter than the Maltese. I prefer that.'

We walked further along Racecourse Street to reach a small market square, before turning up a steep, narrow road. I was quick to memorise a couple of little bars that I liked the look of, for future investigation.

The Citadel was entered through a gateway set within the massive fortifications. Beyond these great walls, a cathedral basked silent and resplendent in the still warm sunlight. I tugged on Nan's arm and we continued through the ramparts, out of the shade. She had suddenly become quiet, unusually distant.

I counted the steps leading up to the cathedral, and we had

reached number twenty when Nan asked me to stop. Two young boys were crouched playing marbles beside us.

'Wait, Harry.' She appeared worried, and I was surprised to notice her trembling. 'There's something I want you to know.'

'What is it, Nan? Are you all right?' I clutched her against me.

'Yes, fine, I just had a funny feeling.' She looked at me with lost, drowning eyes. I felt her body gradually begin to loosen and relax against my own. 'Harry, I want you to know that I truly love you.'

'I know that, Nan.' I held her away from me, smiling.

'But I will always love you.' She spoke more faintly now, determined. 'As long as I live.'

She pressed her face against my neck, and I never thought that I could be so happy. We had climbed the first twenty steps to my heart. We kissed, again, and it was another ten to reach the building. I glanced up to notice the watchful eye of the Virgin staring down at us from the cathedral facade.

It was a sluggish heat. We explored the cathedral square, where olive trees added a dusty silver to the golden aura of reflected sunlight, and it was possible to look back on Victoria under the archway we had walked through. Nan explained that the Citadel had originally constituted the capital of Gozo, with Victoria a later suburb. It had been chosen for its location, perched on a hill overlooking both the city and island. She had recovered quickly, returning to her usual animated self.

A few buildings remained intact behind the cathedral, but much of the ground was littered with yellow stone rubble. Tumbledown walls, almond trees, and prickly pears were abundant. With every few steps, haughty lizards scuttled out of our way, their heads held high from the ground. Despite this sense of abandonment, the Citadel climbed unequivocally majestic into a sky without clouds. There was something heroic about it.

It was possible to gain access onto the ramparts, and to walk around these battlements. Nan was worried that I might act foolhardily, and walk too close to the edge, but there was little chance of this. I clutched her hand tightly, a fear of heights preventing any desire to approach and look down at the sheer drop.

Seven flat-topped hills sprung up from a green patchwork of fields, and I could see a distant strip of deep blue Mediterranean in every direction. This pleased me. Noises from the country floated up to us, of tinkling goat bells, the bleating of sheep, a madness of church bells. Between these conic hills, low ridges had been formed which enclosed the larger villages and towns. Buildings shone as white as newly hatched eggs. The Citadel cast a great, lengthening shadow over the fields far below.

I found myself drawn to the eastern wall, directly behind the cathedral. Here, it was possible to make out Mgarr harbour in the distance, Comino, and Malta. Nan pointed out the towns of Marsalforn, Xewkija, and Xlendi, where we planned to visit. From our high vantage point, the countryside appeared ribboned with tiny grey roads, houses relatively scarce. We stayed here for a long time, sitting on the stone wall, and watched the sun set behind us making the church at San Lawrenz glow as if on fire. It remained a wonderful prospect to be on holiday together, and to be allowed to rest properly after all that had transpired.

Nan and I were the only guests in the hotel dining room

that first evening. To my surprise and delight, she wore her white dress from the dance at the hospital. I hadn't realised she had packed it. Her hair was allowed to fall loose and she never used make-up. She had no need of this.

Noel seated us in the middle of a candle-lit room, our table decorated with peonies. I ordered a bottle of the local red wine, although Nan preferred to drink lemonade. Two brands were available on the island, and it amused me that she would only ever touch the Lighthouse variety. It was produced on Castle Street, next to the Citadel, and she said that it reminded her of our meeting and first kiss in Valletta. The bottle was a proper work of art, a jaunty blue lighthouse painted onto white glass.

The food served by Noel was fantastic. He brought us a selection of local peppered cheese and tomatoes before our starters of minestrone soup. I had a whole silver bream, stuffed with onion and tomato, and Nan ate her first Lampuki pie for years. The bread, fish, and vegetables, were of a quality I had never experienced, the wine as good as Nan's prediction. Noel made sure that my glass was never allowed to empty, and I noticed how he would catch any loose drops with a practised flick of his little finger against the bottle, so preventing crimson stain on the pristine white tablecloth.

It's the tomatoes I most remember, for they were a strange, elongated shape, as if stuffed through a tube although certainly not a sigmoidoscope. They tasted unbelievable, like some exotic fruit. It seemed that we had been hungry for years, and we ate greedily, catching up for lost opportunity.

I continued to make Nan laugh, borrowing jokes from Dicky Fuller and relating incidents from my nurse training.

With each fresh eruption and shake of the head, her hair swept over her face, and she repositioned this delicately behind each ear. She smiled often, eyes shining brightly, and I remained as much in awe of her beauty as when we had first met. We held hands, our legs entwined beneath the table, and decided to retire early to bed.

Drawing back the shutters in the morning, I discovered a world that had turned to silver. The early light and a fine mist had conspired to paint a magical vision, affecting both the gardens and neighbouring houses. All was silent. It was too beautiful to keep to myself.

I woke Nan with a kiss on the mouth. She sat in front of me on the floor, my arms and legs wrapped about her naked body. I loved her smell in the mornings, and was able to kiss her neck, to bury my face into her hair. She responded by leaning backwards, and we remained braided together until the sun eventually managed to burn through, flooding colour into the day. I continued to feel charmed, that nothing could or would go wrong.

Our bathroom was located at the end of the corridor, the towels provided by the hotel barely adequate to cover a single buttock. I felt so light-hearted, elated, that I decided to jog naked along the passageway.

'Come on, Nan!'

There had been no sign of any fellow guests, and I skipped from the room with a towel resting over my shoulder. My face must have been a picture when three doors suddenly opened, to allow their occupants out.

There was only one thing to do; I continued on my way, feigning nonchalance. I walked calmly, wishing everybody a 'Good Morning', and it seemed even then to be one of the big moments in my life. I would not have changed a thing. I could not have felt greater contentment, and Nan's laughter filled me with hope for our future. One of the male guests gestured that she should follow my example, an offer Nan was quick to decline.

Breakfast was as good as the evening meal, with Noel again on duty. He brought us omelettes, a selection of fruit, and freshly squeezed orange juice produced from trees in the hotel courtyard. Noel said that they all worked hard on the island, many people having two jobs. A couple of guests nodded wryly in my direction, and I smiled cheerfully back.

'I've always had this thing about eggs, Nan.' My mind wandered. 'Ever since I was a child, I've been afraid that one day I'll find a chick inside. Even now, the thought still gets me.'

'Harry, I think I need to explain some stuff to you.' She placed one hand over mine. 'Have you ever heard about fertilisation? No? After breakfast, you can have your lesson.' Her fingers gripped tight, entwining between my own.

We decided to explore Victoria. Nan and I meandered through a maze of narrow streets, some no more than six feet wide, where it was easy to remain in the shade. Statues of the Virgin adorned many buildings and street corners, clutching the baby Jesus, and Nan smiled in their acknowledgement. The majority of houses formed long terraces, plain two-storey affairs made handsome by elegant, ornate balconies. A sea of blue-green filigree and shadows danced blithely over our heads.

We walked slowly, always touching, along cool, winding streets leading into charming little squares, each of them different. Trees appeared to be growing everywhere, unusual after Malta, and I recognised one bar from the previous evening. The Café de la Reine looked particularly inviting, with a hushed, dark interior. A murmur of foreign voices drifted out through the open door and I was ready for a beer. I asked Nan if she wanted to go in, but she turned down this suggestion.

'Women don't go into bars, Harry. Not just to drink.'

It had not been like this on Malta.

It was quiet in Victoria, relatively deserted, and I found this suited me. On Gozo, it seemed that we were not only outside the war, but also outside of time. Nan and I had stumbled into a place where we could live forever, everything else in our lives faded from view. There were no complications. It was an exhilarating sensation, almost tangible, with anything remaining possible between us.

We passed groups of old men smoking blackened pipes, twisted and bent, as gnarled as old trees. Others sat alone in shaded doorways, lost to their thoughts, wearing little black caps. They nodded at us from well-worn steps, occasionally accompanied by silent women sewing intricate patterns of lace.

Back at the hotel, Noel was able to tell me about the war on the island. I questioned him while enjoying a bottle of Blue Label. Nan was upstairs, soaking in a bath.

'It wasn't so bad here, sir.'

'Call me Harry.'

He smiled, carefully polishing glasses behind the long, wooden bar. A shiny brass fan whirred above our heads.

'We were unprotected, but escaped most of the bombing. Of course there were a few raids. Nadur took a bad hit, as did Sannat. But we were lucky compared to you. Where were you based?'

'M'tarfa, at the hospital. And Nan was in Valletta for a good while.'

'So you saw the worst of it then. And the hunger - we didn't have any real food shortages on Gozo.'

'Thanks for sending us the wheat.'

Noel looked up from his work and smiled again. We had the dining room to ourselves, and I looked through the windows at the adjacent gardens where a scrawny black cat stared defiantly back.

'Many Maltese came here, for safety,' he continued. 'That changed the island. It was too busy, and I'm glad most of them have gone home. But they used to put on shows for us, here in Victoria.'

'We had ENSA, some of it was good. Do you think it will all soon be over, Noel?'

'I hope so, sir.' He turned to replace the glasses onto their respective shelves. 'I hope so.'

Our travels took us all over the island. We had both packed lightly, through necessity, and Nan favoured a particular dress for our walking excursions. It was the clear blue of the sea, decorated with tiny sunflowers, fitting closely over her curves. She carried a floppy straw hat that always dipped at the front.

We ventured to the west coast, beginning our journey through Victoria. In one square, not far from the hotel, several old ladies sat gathered on rickety wooden chairs outside an enormous church. It had the same twin towers as those on Malta. These ladies trilled noisily and Nan released my hand, walking over to join their conservation. I followed slowly, able only to stand and watch, eyeing a nearby bar and considering a Blue Label beer.

Nan appeared to become upset, shaking her head vigorously, raising her voice. She sounded so different when speaking in Maltese, invariably louder. I watched her legs cross over each other, something she always did when agitated.

'What was that about?'

She returned to my side with tears in her eyes. I took her hand and we resumed our walk.

'The war again, Harry. That's what they were talking about. I asked them how it had been.'

'Noel was telling me last night.'

'You never said?' She glanced at me.

'We had other things to talk about. Better things.'

We had been reminiscing about our years together, those stolen nights in Buskett Gardens and the field outside Mdina. Nan had said how she was worried that I would prefer going out in Strait Street, but she had quickly realised otherwise. I didn't want to share her at all; our time together was far better spent when alone.

'Anyway, they were telling me about a bomb that hit Sannat. One of these women lost a sister, and her daughter. She was only one, Harry, fast asleep in a hammock. She died two days later, from internal injuries. It's dreadful.' Nan spoke with tired anger. 'And then I asked what had been damaged the most.'

She shook her head again. 'They told me that the Americans had pulled down the Gourgion Tower outside Xewkija. It wasn't even bombed - they knocked it down to build a runway, and now its hardly ever used! I went there before, Harry, and it was so beautiful. I can't really believe it. It's these things that make me want to cry.'

She began to sob. I held Nan against me, her hair in my face, one hand pressing on the small of her back. I kissed her head, squeezing her tightly. It made me love her even more, and I had not believed that was possible.

The road carried us past fields ripe with plump watermelons napping in the sunlight, looking like nothing I'd ever seen before. I swear I saw an old woman with a full beard, sitting in shade at the side of the road; I hadn't seen that, either. There were owners who looked like their dogs, little birds darting into nests hidden within old stone walls, and tiny houses that could only hold dwarves. My room and window in the barracks was made to seem palatial. Horses rested in back yards, with fig trees, fennel, and capers lining the roadside.

People stopped us at regular intervals, questioning our wisdom to walk. We were told that it was too hot, too far, sheer madness, although Gozo is a small island. The sun poured down, relentless, but our pace remained good and strong. With Nan at my side, together, I continued to feel invincible.

Through the village of San Lawrenz, we stumbled down a steep dirt track cursed with numerous hairpin bends.

'That's the Fungus Rock, over there.' Nan pointed to an inlet where a lonely cliff stood perpendicular out of the milky-blue water. It dropped straight into a white curl of sea foam, and was topped with a dark green covering.

'What's that?' My feet skidded on loose stone at the side of the road.

'It's famous. It used to be guarded because of the fungus that grows on the surface. It's very rare, Harry, supposed to have excellent healing properties, especially for bleeding and dysentery.' Nan brushed hair from her face, walking quickly now. Our feet made a satisfying crunch on the gravel.

'You mean like I had?'

'Yes! Like that!' She squeezed my hand, smiling at me.

'Well I wish they'd given me some of that instead of the damn sigmoidoscope!'

Nan burst into laughter.

The track twisted right as we approached the sea, a massive rock archway becoming visible over the water. It resembled a giant stone door, complete with lintel, set into the cliff face. The sea beneath this arch appeared the refined blue of a rich man's swimming pool.

'And what's that?' I felt like an inquisitive child, bursting with questions.

'The Azure Window. It's impressive, yes?'

We clambered over rocks to enjoy a closer view. The sea was calm, resembling a giant lake, and still it roared in my ears. I always liked it when it did that. Nan removed her hat, releasing her hair to blow free.

'You're right. Gozo's lovely.'

I took her in my arms, our lips meeting instinctively, willing time to forget about us. To leave us alone. I understood all too well how being with Nan was my fate, my intended path in life. Not for me was the drudgery of England, a dull, monotonous existence; I was born to another direction, one that separated me from the others. At that moment, I came to accept this, to rejoice in it. We had a future and it was here, something that had never been discussed. If only I dared to voice it. It was a road that nobody else had trodden, a remarkable thing, and I held onto Nan saying nothing. Her eyes remained closed while I stared into the distance, my gaze beyond the water. I don't know why I remained silent.

A short walk brought us to the Inland Sea. The lime green water was actually a small lake connected with the Mediterranean through a natural rock tunnel. Nan said that dolphins occasionally strayed into the bay, needing help to return to sea. A small café was present, where we sat under cover from the sun. I finally had my Blue Label beer, and Nan her Lighthouse lemonade. She insisted that we share a salad, so keeping us both happy. Little fish were visible in the shallow water near to our feet. Boathouses had been hewn out of the cliffs to our right. We sat close, bare legs touching beneath a wobbly iron table, listening to the tender swirl of the sea.

A definite highlight of the holiday was being able to share a bed, with early nights fast becoming a priority. I would curl myself into her, groin wedged against her bottom, one arm resting over both breasts. If I should turn over, Nan would press fiercely against me, her heat burning into me, and in this way we were able to sleep as one.

I adored the lazy sweetness of our mornings. We slept deeply, undisturbed. The days flew past like butterflies, and here I dreamed only of colours. If I should wake first, I would sit carefully upright, watching Nan while she slept. Her features softened, breathing easy. Her eyelashes flickered gently as I tried to count them.

After she woke, we talked and invariably loved. Nan lay face down, stretched out luxuriously, and I straddled her warm body. I ran my hands firmly from her shoulders, up her neck, across her back, and over her bottom. I listened to her sighs and little groans, and then I changed position. I worked my hands down long legs to her feet, enjoying the smooth, firm touch of her skin. We loved slowly, unhurried, with all the time in the world. Whenever Nan moved from the bed, I buried my face into her pillow, inhaling her musky perfume with deep breaths. I positioned myself carefully onto the heat she had left behind.

Noel arranged a couple of bicycles for us, to explore the island more thoroughly. We saw the Neolithic temples at Xaghra, the windmill at Qala, a wild sea galloping and stamping hoof marks onto the saltpans near Zebbug. At Marsalforn, we saw two girls on a balcony dancing into the sunset. One wore a white slip, the second a red one, both of them swinging breasts and hips like church bells with a jubilant sense of abandon. The sun cast an orange net over the sea, a solitary white cloud stretched into a straight line until it was also changed to orange. Everyone we met on the island appeared to be happy, content with their lot, secure in the knowledge that living here they were onto a good thing.

It became routine for Nan and me to visit the Citadel each evening, before returning to the hotel. We sat and gazed over the country, usually from the east wall, and this was my favourite view of Gozo. It had been an unspoken agreement between us that we should never discuss the future, our life after the war, but one week into the holiday it was Nan who changed the rules. The sun was beginning to set behind us, the sky striated with deep bands of red.

'I like it when it's quiet, like this.' She spoke softly, deliberately. 'I would love to travel the world, to see England, but I want to live here. I don't want to leave.' Nan glanced towards me before turning slowly, surveying the city below.

'There are not so many cars. You can walk or catch a ride anywhere. The people are good. It's beautiful. And safe. Yes, I want to stay here.'

I remained silent, my heart beating rapidly. Nan could have been reading my mind; I did not want to leave Gozo.

'After the war, I would like to start painting again. Maybe even teach art. I could be on the Citadel every day - it would be wonderful.' A ghost of a smile touched her face, her lips pursed thoughtfully together.

'I didn't know you painted, Nan?'

She moved to face me, one hand resting onto my leg. 'I'm just a beginner really, but the teacher said I was good. We started by copying scenes - things like Christmas trees on cards, which I wasn't so keen on. But I would like to try - how do you call it – abstract. Yes. It looks easy, but this is not so.' She paused, swallowing. 'Would you join me here, Harry?'

'Yes.' It was the question I'd been waiting and hoping for. My heart blazed with joy, tears instantly filling my eyes. 'Of course I would. Yes!'

She touched my face, now smiling. 'We can make many babies, and live in the sunshine.'

'I'd love it, Nan. No more cold England, and plenty of Blue Label beer!'

'You!' She pushed a hand against my chest.

'Really, it would be wonderful. I'd love to. They'll always need nurses, so maybe I could work in the hospital.'

'So it's agreed, then?' She held out her hand.

'It's agreed.'

In this way, we shook hands on our future together.

CHAPTER SEVENTEEN

After the war, I was out with Eric Reynolds. Gwen and Elsie Galey were meeting us later, in Shepherds Bush, and we were drinking in the Hambone Club. The room was layered with thick bands of smoke. I had my hand in a bowl of peanuts, and Eric was telling me about his latest conquest. Women were always propositioning him, and it happened so rarely to me. I listened with envy and admiration.

'So how's it going with Gwen, then? Are you back to breaking those bed springs?'

I was living with Gwen. It was terrible. How could I have left Nan? It made no sense. I woke panting, sitting upright, splashing to the surface of consciousness.

I glanced about the room. Nan was sleeping beside me, stirring at the disturbance, and I was back in the Duke of Edinburgh Hotel. Thank God, it was all a dream. A nightmare. I vowed that would never happen to me; it was much too awful a prospect. When Nan opened her eyes, I kissed her on the lips. She responded by pulling me down, to lie by her side.

'I like waking up with you, Harry. Don't ever leave me.'

'I'm not,' I answered. 'I'm not going anywhere.'

Our favourite place on the island became Xlendi Bay, on the south coast. It was a half-hour walk from Victoria, through a valley crammed with almond, olive, and carob trees. Birdsong prettied the air, small churches dotting the horizon. The usual pink and white oleanders bordered the roadside.

We passed through the village of Fontana, where tiny, wrinkled old ladies could always be seen laundering their clothes in an old stone washhouse. It was positioned over a natural spring, the water virgin pure. Nan always shouted out greetings, chuckling to herself.

'The fights that happen here, Harry,' she whispered. 'You wouldn't believe it. Woe betide the woman who uses her neighbour's space - she's really in for it!'

The old ladies nodded and smiled sweetly at our passing.

The road dipped sharply on entering Xlendi, with fields stretching right down to the sea. A scattering of houses was present, a sandy beach, the bay itself a long, narrow cove sheltered by steep cliffs on either side.

'You've got to see this, Harry.' Nan tugged on my arm, pulling me towards the sheer climb of a cliff face.

'What is it?'

'Another secret place, like at Dingli.'

Stone steps appeared, carved crudely into the rock, leading to a cave with only lizards for company. This fed into a hidden bathing spot, where white sand caused the water to shine a brilliant emerald green.

'Look! It's the colour of your eyes. I always knew they reminded me of something.' Nan was delighted. 'The nuns used to come here for privacy Harry, to protect their modesty,' she laughed.

This fact had an overpowering, strange effect on me. There was not a soul around, I was with the woman I loved, and we were in a place haunted by naked nuns. Into that green water, I undressed and walked without hesitation. Nan followed. Right here, we enjoyed making slow, tender, love.

As we returned along the steps, scrambling up into the sunlight, a large white butterfly fluttered into sight. It proceeded to follow Nan whether she walked, ran, or stood still, remaining with her until we reached the beach. A similar thing had happened at Marsaxlokk. I could make no sense to this, but it felt like another good omen, somehow consolidating the happiness that we enjoyed. Nan said that it was probably her guardian angel. My shoes were discarded, and I jumped onto the hot sand of the beach, digging words into the strand. '*I Love Nan*'.

The water was incredibly buoyant, perfect for swimming, and we were able to dive from rocks opposite the hidden cave. I slipped once, falling in like an idiot, and true to form I lost my shorts on one particular high dive. We were in and out of the water all day, Nan by far the stronger swimmer. While I floated on my back, content to sunbathe, she swam swift lengths across the bay.

My hair had grown like a weed in the heat, becoming increasingly curly without its weekly trim, and the seawater thankfully helped to control this. I preferred it cropped short but Nan had professed to love it, constantly playing with her hands through its lengthening locks. If it made her happy, then I was prepared to let it grow wild.

In Xlendi, I saw colours that I had never witnessed elsewhere, ranging from green to gold to scarlet and red. We watched a bright orange sun set down the exact centre of the cove, the water at night becoming milky white. Shooting stars lit up the sky on the walk back to Victoria, the cicadas singing lustily. Little bats swooped and darted joyfully, aiming straight for us, before glancing away at the very last moment. The air remained warm, scented with exotic perfumes, while behind us the sea removed all trace of my words, renouncing their message of love.

It was on the way to Ta Pinu, to visit the church, that we finally accepted a ride. Nan was wearing her sunflower dress, the air especially balmy, and it seemed churlish to refuse the kind farmer who stopped his donkey-pulled cart for us to climb into the back.

The sky was a perfect blue. Fields speckled with tomatoes trundled past, an aqueduct pacing the land to our left. Nan seemed particularly excited.

'You must see this place, Harry. You'll love it. It's a very important church.'

The roads were empty. Most people took shelter until the relative cool of evening, and the heat was now intense. Nan put on her hat. Butterflies danced intricate routines in the sky above our heads.

'Why here, Nan?' There were countless churches on Gozo, as there had been on Malta.

'An old peasant woman lived nearby. Karmela Grima. She was working in the fields, and heard the Madonna's voice. Right here.'

'When?'

'1883. Harry, what was it you used to say? 'Ask me another one!' I know all about this. It's a place of miracles. Look, there it is!'

A large isolated chapel came into view in front of us, awkward in its surroundings. It was certainly grand, built on an impressive scale, but I wouldn't have realised it was anything special. All of the island's churches seemed lavish to me.

'There's Karmela Grima's house.' Nan pointed to an oppressive stone building with tiny windows. It looked more like a prison, and I wondered if the voice she heard had anything to do with light deprivation and a temporary madness. 'They built this church around the old one, Harry, and people come here on pilgrimage. You must pray here. It's a custom to leave things after Our Lady has listened, you'll see, we call it ex-votos.' She grasped both my hands in earnest, insistent. 'You must pray here, Harry, it will be answered.'

Our driver slowed to a halt, waving goodbye. 'Come on,' Nan shouted, jumping from the cart, impatient to enter the building. I followed close behind, admiring her figure as usual, and keen to escape from the sun.

A deep silence flowed into the church. Nan crossed herself before walking slowly forwards, beckoning I should follow. Two women sat praying, facing the altar, but Nan led me into a side room where photographs lined the walls, along with typed letters and scribbled prayers of people cured from illness. There were old crutches and plaster casts no longer required, fishing line that had saved lives, baby clothes thankfully grown out of, against all odds. 'You see?' Nan murmured, taking my hand and returning to the chapel. She crossed herself once more, before kneeling in front of a rather solemn Virgin. Unsure how to act, I copied and fell to my own knees.

The stone of the floor was cold, and I rested back on my haunches. To my amazement I found myself praying, unbidden words streaming up into the sky, emerging naked from deep inside. I prayed to the Lady of Ta Pinu that our love would never die, that only death could keep us apart. I gave thanks for finding the woman who understood me so completely, for the happiness that we experienced. I hoped that it should be able to continue. I prayed that the future we had agreed upon should be allowed to happen, that we could both find work and remain on the island. I prayed that we should one day have a family.

I opened my eyes and raised my head, looking up to the

face of the icon. A sense of deliverance filled my body, excitement, the hairs on my arms and neck stood up in recognition. I knew that the Lady had listened, my prayers received and taken notice. Everything would be all right, given time. Nan's family would come to accept me. We would have those children, a boy and a girl. When I turned around, I realised that I kneeled on my own. Nan stood waiting for me outside.

At the hotel, in our room, it was Nan who wrote on my back 'I will always love you', retracing her Egyptian eye to ward off evil spirits. I rested my head on the skin of her stomach, listening to the secret sounds within, willing myself to fuse into her. For us to become as one.

We visited Sannat, the red sandy beach of Ramla Bay, the colourful fields outside Nadur. This island seemed like paradise. On the penultimate night, I left Nan sleeping in bed; it was hotter than usual. I needed some air, and wanted time to think on my own.

It was not late, maybe ten, but the streets of Victoria were already empty of people. Even the busy Café de la Reine was closed, and it seemed as if the world had stopped turning. All around me was darkness and silence, as if I was the last man on earth, and this felt surprisingly good. I climbed onto the ramparts of the Citadel, and to my favourite spot on the east wall. I could see nothing, the moon hidden with cloud, and I began to consider the future.

I believed in many things: duty, responsibility, and to some degree fate. But the thing I believed in most was the undeniable force and power of love. The prospect of any future had to include Nan. There was simply no choice about this.

Gwen would be all right, she was a survivor. She had

coped after Clem, her husband, deserted her, and I felt certain that my own disappearance would bring about a fleeting annoyance, nothing more. I had sent her the bulk of my wages from the time spent on Malta, but she was a woman who would always find money from somewhere.

It would be harder to leave my family, especially mother. Lilian had always been so good and kind, I felt sure that she would understand my departure, but it pained me all the same. Father I would miss less, but his health suffered badly. I hoped to see him one last time, that we might make up and become friends. I hoped he would be proud of my army service.

Would I miss England? London, yes. Folkestone, probably not. I hadn't lived there for years. I was swimming deeper and deeper into such thoughts when an even stronger idea crashed through to reach me. Nan was alone, asleep in our bed. Naked. It did not take long to run back to the Duke of Edinburgh, and I only fell the once.

Our last day was touched with a definite sadness. We visited Xlendi, swimming in a sea that shimmered blue as the summer sky. We wandered slowly through Fontana, past the washhouse, before eventually returning to Victoria. Sitting on the edge of the ramparts, under a still fierce sun, I wound a finger into Nan's hair. She rested against me, and we looked towards the port of Mgarr and Malta.

'Goodbye Citadel. Goodbye Gozo.' She whispered the words. It was a daunting prospect to be leaving. These had been the best two weeks of my life, and I feared already that the future could not remain as good. We had been cocooned on this little island, undisturbed and untouched by all outside events.

We waited until the sun had disappeared before turning

and walking slowing along the walls, then back down steps leading into Victoria. I could now identify for myself the town of Xewkija, Sannat hanging by fingertips onto the edge of a cliff, the plump, cosy harbour at Marsalforn, and I wondered how long it would be before we were allowed to return. Words seemed somehow indecent. I could hear a car horn sound frantically from far away, the distant noise of everyday life to which we returned with reluctance. The future disturbed both our thoughts.

I settled up with Noel and presented him a generous tip. Service and food in the hotel had been fantastic.

'Thank you Harry, it's been a pleasure.' He did not look to check how much money I placed into his hand. 'You'll be coming back to see us?'

'I hope so. Will you still be here?'

He smiled, shaking my hand with genuine warmth. 'It's my dream to be wearing a white shirt and black trousers at the age of sixty, God willing.' He gestured with his hands. 'I want to have people nod at me in recognition, saying to each other, 'Look, the old waiter is still here.''

'Well I wish you all the best, Noel.'

It was only after we'd left, rolling away in a karozzin, that I realised he'd called me Harry. It was the first time, despite my many protests. I stuck my head though the carriage window and smiled. Noel remained waving outside the hotel, making broad sweeps in the air with his right arm.

The fishing boat took us back a different way, sailing around the far side of Comino. Vertical cliffs stood like castle walls, a heap of boulders visible at the sea edge. It was only then that I realised we had never made it to the Blue Lagoon.

CHAPTER EIGHTEEN

There had been no new cases of polio at the hospital. The outbreak was definitely over. All admissions were the usual mixture of diarrhoeas and dysenteries, easily managed, and life on the ward ticked over nicely. Olivia Merciecp had proven an able deputy, and I slipped quietly back into my duties. It was difficult, I was used to being with Nan.

The paperwork was up to date, and supplies now arrived regularly on the island. The shortages of soap, medicine, and food, were quickly forgotten, making it much easier to care for our patients. Laughter had returned to F Block and the barracks, a general sense of optimism.

It was during the first week back at work that Matron rushed into the ward late one afternoon. I was sitting at the desk, pretending to be busy, and remembering the two girls dancing on the balcony at Marsalforn. The way they had moved, arms held high in the air, was really something. You couldn't help but smile at their exultation, and I had raised a glass of Blue Label in their honour. They had spotted Nan and me, the only people on the promenade, and danced especially for us. When Matron strolled up to the desk, she took me quite by surprise.

'Harold, you've got to come with me. Sister Merciecp can look after the ward.'

'What is it Matron?' I was amazed to see her hair released from its normal stranglehold, flowing in luxuriant waves down her back, rippling like dark water. Matron was smiling, possibly even wearing lipstick, and looked a good ten years younger than usual.

'I can't tell you, but it's excellent news. Come on, the

Major's waiting for you in his office.' She tapped her heels impatiently.

We walked from the building into the heat of the gardens. It was quiet outside, except for the resident cicadas. The figs on the tree beside F Block looked nearly ready for eating, if the birds didn't get there first. The oleanders were in constant pink and white bloom.

Matron refused to divulge any information, insisting only that we should hurry. I struggled to keep pace and when we reached the hospital reception, she patted me on my way.

'He's waiting upstairs, you don't need me to go with you. I'll see you later Harold, I'm so pleased.' She continued to beam.

'Can't you tell me anything?' I called over my shoulder.

'Go and talk to the Major,' came her reply.

The door to his office stood open and he was pacing the tiny room manically, stiff arms jerking like metronomes. There was only sufficient space for two strides in either direction.

'Harold,' he noticed my arrival. 'You've made it!' The Major was chuckling to himself, spectacles sitting on the desk, and I wondered what was happening. Had the world gone mad in my absence? 'Come here, well done!' He shook my hand enthusiastically, one arm wrapping briefly about my shoulders. The man was making me nervous.

'What is it Major?'

'Henry, please. Call me Henry,' he interrupted. 'It's great news isn't it, Harold? Well done!'

'What is, Maj-' I stopped myself. 'Henry?' The word felt unnatural in my mouth. It was easier, far preferable, to stick to our normal relations. 'Nobody has told me anything.'

'You mean you don't know?' he exploded a laugh of

amazement. 'That's even better, it means I get to tell you.' He had kept hold of my hand, and now began shaking it again. Vigorously. His face was flushed beetroot red.

'You've got the British Empire Medal, my man! From now on, it's Harold Fisher BEM. And I'm an MBE. It's excellent, isn't it?'

'Yes. I suppose it is.' All I wanted was to find Nan, to hold her, to share this information. I was imagining her reaction when the Major continued to speak.

'The Colonels pass on their thanks, Morrison and Harding. They said it was only through our combined skills and hard work that the death roll was kept so low. Well done, Harold!' Finally, he released my hand, bending to the drawer of his desk. 'Can I offer you a whisky?'

I met Nan in the courtyard outside my quarters as darkness began to fall. We walked quickly to our field, the sky mushroomed with red, and only then I told her my news. She screamed in excited delight, jumping on the spot, fists clenched, her arms raised up to the sky.

'Harry, that's wonderful! I can't tell you how proud I am.'

'Can't you try?' I grabbed her about the waist, and she screamed right into my ear. 'On second thoughts, maybe not.'

Nan wore her brown dress, one that was easily removed. Tonight it was a frantic type of love and, after, we lay exhausted and sweaty on top of our discarded clothes. I kissed her face, her breasts, her thighs.

'So do you think it will make it any easier for me to stay on the island?'

'I hope so,' she pulled me hard against her. 'But I know my family will definitely be impressed.'

We remained outside all night.

A party was held in my honour in the Sergeants' Mess. It was a decent turn out for a weekday night, and the alcohol flowed freely. Our personal allocation had gone up after the siege, increased to one bottle of whisky per week. Somebody had borrowed a wind-up gramophone, and the voice of Vera Lynn struggled to be heard above the sound of the men. Unfortunately, Victory V cigarettes were again plentiful on the island, ensuring the room was hazy with smoke. I popped outside for some much needed fresh air when Dicky Fuller appeared from out of nowhere.

'All right Harry, how you doing?' He smiled. 'I wanted to say goodbye.'

'How come Dicky? I'm glad you've made it.' I had gone to considerable trouble to make sure an invitation reached him.

'They're sending me home, Harry.' Dicky slapped me on the back. 'Back to bloody Folkestone.'

'But why?'

'Don't need me out here any more.' He wasn't joking. It was the only time I had heard him arrive anywhere without laughter. 'I'll miss the old place. So see you at home, eh?'

'Aren't you coming inside, to the party?'

'Sorry mate, I'm not in the mood. Got to pack and I'm off first thing in the morning.'

I could understand exactly how he felt. We embraced and he disappeared into the darkness. I returned to Mess with the firm intention of getting drunk as quickly as possible, countless bottles of Blue Label emptied down my throat. The occasion did not feel like a celebration any more.

'Hello Harold.' Major Merryweather pushed through to join me, his glasses all steamed up. I hadn't been expecting to see him; he had his own party to attend. We shook hands.

I attempted a grin while trying hard to act sober.

'Thanks Major Henry.'

He smiled. 'It's been a long haul, hasn't it? Four years now. But you deserve this. Wanted to show my face.'

'Nearly. Nearly Four.' I remembered this date from the anniversary of meeting with Nan. A drunken chorus of *White Cliffs of Dover* began mauling its way about the room.

'Shouldn't think it will be long now. Our paths have followed each other so far Harold, you never know, we might see each other back in England?'

'Yes.' I hoped not. I had no intention of leaving. A drink was pressed into my hand and someone slapped me on the back. 'Well, cheers!'

The contents were downed in a single gulp, to the obvious dismay of the Major. He shook his head frantically, grabbing at my arm, attempting to make me stop.

'You don't want to drink that, Harold. Damn beer's been spiked with whisky.'

It was the last thing I remembered.

I woke in my clothes. The room was still dark and it hurt to swallow, my throat sandpapered raw. This was nothing compared to the pain behind my eyes, radiating into both temples. The moment I moved, I knew I was going to be sick. But I didn't have control of my limbs, and threw up all over my clothes. My nose must have been the only part of me that was unaffected, because it smelt dreadful. And I was used to the odour of dysentery.

I fell out of bed, realising immediately that I was going to be sick again. I grabbed the nearest receptacle and threw up extravagantly into my shoe. This was not a good start to the day. I had to crawl to the washroom, where I think I must have passed out. When I next opened my eyes, white light poked needles into both retinas. I was sick again, but couldn't be bothered to move.

It was a shell of a man who eventually arrived on F Block. My insides hurt from repeated retching when there was nothing left to produce, my mouth stung with the taste of bile. I probably stank, but Olivia Merciecp managed to appear pleased to see me.

'Oh Harold, we were so worried" she ran to my side, helping me to sit at the desk.

'Sorry, Olivia, probably made a fool of myself.' My tongue felt swollen, sticking dry to the back of my palate.

'But you went missing, Matron told me. They had to send out a search party.' Olivia now let out a giggle, clutching one hand in front of her mouth, and I groaned more from embarrassment than pain. 'They said they found you back at the barracks, in bed, and snoring like a bastard.'

Nan and I continued to walk to Buskett Gardens whenever possible, and to the cove at Dingli cliffs. The ground in the gardens had become corrugated where we lay, mirroring the underside of our mat, and I was pleased to leave this mark. It struck me as something tangible, proof of our time together. Circling white butterflies continued to visit us, and Nan had shown me how to cut open a prickly pear. The fruit was succulent inside, the flesh sweet and juicy.

The days remained hot, and it was good to be able to swim. The cove was always deserted. After we emerged from the sea, Nan would lie on top of me, stretched along the length of my body. I was aware of her heart thudding strong and sure against my own, saltwater dripping from her body and over me. I imagined osmosis of our beings, invisible threads stretching out from the surface of our skins to link us together, and I felt reluctant to move, to avoid disrupting this bond. Touching my lips across her mouth, cheek, neck, the ends of her hair, I was always aware of the press of her breasts against my sternum. I imagined the blood racing throughout my body detouring into Nan, her own tiny corpuscles entering into me.

We spent most of our off-duty time together, and fate continued to smile upon us. Only rarely this proved impossible. On such occasions I ventured into Valletta, but it was not the same without Dicky Fuller. The magic of the place had gone, the capital now reduced to a bunch of bars crowded with drunken fools and sherry bandits.

Groups of men and women swarmed along the Gut, giddy with a sense of imminent liberation. Soldiers continued to fall in love six times a night and the women were out in force, but I was never unfaithful to Nan. I was never tempted. There were shouts and toasts to good old Blighty, conversations always returned to home, and there was only so much of it that I could take. I walked alone, passing time at the viewpoint on Fountain Street, considering myself the one and only soldier who hoped to remain on the island. There was nothing for me in England.

The radio continued to prove popular on F Block, and we still listened to the broadcasts of Winston Churchill. News from the war was good, and victory had begun to seem inevitable. With Italy out of the fighting, our troops now surged through Europe in pursuit of retreating Jerry. Patients appeared to recover from illness more quickly, their eyes now bright and alert. The prevailing atmosphere in the Gut mirrored this sense of optimism.

It was not long into these hard-earned days of celebration that a telegram was delivered to the hospital. I sat completing paperwork garnered from the ward round, and was surprised to notice the official stamp of the King. The envelope was addressed to H.E. Fisher BEM, the writing small and hard, impenetrable black. Reading quickly, I was summoned to meet with the Colonel in Valletta, a car would be sent to collect me at 15.00 hours. I was to be ready and waiting outside the hospital entrance.

The shift finished at 13.00 hours, and I dashed back to barracks both puzzled and excited by this message. Perhaps the Colonel wanted to congratulate me in person on the recent commendation, or there was a promotion possible in the hospital. Several positions had recently become vacant, and the Major had said that my work had been recognised. I took a shower and shaved for the second time that day, greasing my hair meticulously. My uniform was made presentable; I had never been summoned before.

Standing under the silver shade of an olive tree, the car arrived punctually. The driver was a taciturn man, asking only for confirmation of my name, but that was fine with me. I didn't feel like talking. He drove slowly, carefully, taking a long route into Valletta that detoured through the town of Mosta. The day was a hot one, our windows open, but I was already sweating profusely when he dropped me off opposite the Services Club. Armed soldiers stood on guard either side of a wide stone doorway, barring entrance into the palace courtyard beyond.

A man appeared from inside the building, his pale complexion obviously unused to the sunlight, probably new to the island. He wore an immaculate white suit. He was tiny.

'Fisher? For the Colonel?' He spoke in a squeaky voice. 'Come this way.'

The soldiers stood aside and I hurried after this suit. There were palm trees in the courtyard, an old gas lamp, a statue that caught my eye of some man holding a trident, but he veered sharply into the dark passageway, taking care to remain in the shade. He never once checked to see that I followed.

We climbed stone steps hollowed through long years of use, turning left at the top, and heading towards the rear of the building. A line of green doors were firmly shut on either side, no sounds heard from within, and at the end of the corridor we soon reached a dead end. The man tapped twice, rapidly, on the nearest of the doors.

'What is it?' A powerful voice disturbed this claustrophobic hush.

'Fisher here, Colonel,' he squawked. 'Shall I send him in?'

'Yes. Yes. I've been waiting for him.' The voice sounded annoyed, and I cursed my driver for his languidness. If I should be in trouble for arriving late, I would be explaining the reason for this.

The man in the white suit pushed open the door, gesturing that I should enter. He smelled of cologne like Fred, departing with no further words. I walked nervously into a large, shadowed room that was sheltered from the sun by adjacent apartment blocks. An enormous man with a crew-cut lumbered to his feet from behind a desk that overflowed with papers, a row of metallic grey filing cabinets standing to attention behind his back. He stood tall, a monolith in full military uniform. I heard the door click shut, and my heels snapped together in salute. A large, dusty peace lily stood on the floor beside his desk.

'Sit down. Sit down,' he barked. 'I haven't got time for any of this.' He resumed his previous position, and a clock became visible on the wall above his head. Tiny black numbers on a white face announced the time, 15.45 hours.

'So do you know why you are here, Fisher?'

'No, sir. Not at all.' He allowed me to flounder, trapped by the steel of his gaze. 'Is it to do with the commendation?'

'No,' he snorted. I felt heavy drops of sweat drip uncomfortably down both sides. My face began to itch, prickling with sudden heat. The Colonel studied papers on his desk while he continued to speak. 'First, I would like to thank you for all of your work here. I know you've done that well.' I didn't like the emphasis he placed on the end of the sentence, his brusque manner making me anxious. 'But that's not why you're here.' His eyes, narrowed with anger, returned to my face. He snatched at a typed letter with fat, sausage fingers, before brandishing it in the air.

'You have to be packed and ready to return to England by the first available means. I'm not sure exactly when that will be.'

To say that I felt shattered does no justice to the tidal wave of emotions I then experienced. My legs trembled badly beneath the desk. I felt light-headed, and it was a struggle to remain upright. The sweat flowed even more freely now. A pounding began behind my eyes, as destiny was crudely snatched away from me. How could I ever leave Nan?

'We have a letter here, just received, from your dependent's psychiatrist. It states that she is a suicide risk and your return is essential. Take a look, man.'

He shoved the flimsy blue paper across the desk. I bent forwards and picked it up on the second attempt, the words dancing in front of my eyes, refusing to be understood. It took a long moment before I recognised the name of the psychiatrist; he was a close friend and colleague of Gwen.

My return to England was requested in no uncertain terms, in order for our marriage to take place. I read how Gwen was now aged over thirty and desperate to carry our child. If I should not return soon, she would be certain to suffer a nervous breakdown and hence become a suicide risk. It was a crushing, devastating blow, and a total surprise. Gwen had never mentioned any of this in our sporadic correspondence.

'I don't want to leave, sir.' The words were forced with desperation, but too quickly for his liking. Much too quickly.

'I was not offering you a choice, Fisher,' the Colonel shouted. 'Haven't you read the letter? You can forget about your Maltese girlfriend.'

My lungs ground to an asthmatic halt. The blood in my veins stopped flowing, and a sound like the sea roared in my ears, deafening. How did he know about Nan? Who had told him?

'They never settle away from the island, and you're not a damn Catholic. Her family would never accept you.'

The clock turned in silence. At 16.00 hours I was dismissed sharply with orders repeated to leave the island. In fifteen minutes, all my dreams had fractured and broken. I had not realised that a body could experience so much pain until it grew worse, when I saw Nan in the evening.

We had arranged to meet in her quarters. I had never actually been inside, but her roommate had just left and she finally lived on her own. The few blocks separating our rooms might as well have been an ocean that day, and I have no recollection of walking there.

She opened the door, her features radiant with joy. Nan was wearing her lily-white dress, my favourite, but a single glance at me was enough to remove her smile.

'Harry, what is it? What's wrong?' She clutched at my arm, pulling me into the room. I stumbled inside, collapsing to the floor, while Nan closed the door. She moved and sat down to face me, an agony of space between us. Nan bent forwards, grazing my lips with her own, before resting back on her knees. She reached for my hands, our fingers entwining automatically. 'Harry, tell me what it is.'

I looked at her face, those dark eyes, but it was too painful. Her shoulders were bare, uncovered. A tide of golden sunlight washed into the room, casting a halo on the wall above our heads, illuminating the single bed. A white sheet sunk onto the floor, creased like sand dunes in the desert. I told her about the Colonel.

'Our love doesn't have to stop, Harry. Look at me. I've told you that before. I'll always love you.' Her voice sounded so reassuring. My grip tightened in her hands.

'But we won't be together, Nan. It's useless. I don't want to leave you.' I raised my eyes to meet her own.

'I know.' She paused, 'But maybe we have no choice.'

I wanted more than anything for Nan to ask me to stay, to fight for me. I wanted her to save me from myself, and from the future I had stubbornly created back in England. To be both responsible and guilty for me, but most of all I simply wanted her. She had remained calm throughout my news, understanding, almost as if she had prepared for it. Nan possessed the power to make me do anything, but now she was too good.

'I've some bad news too, Harry. There's been an accident at Bari, and they're sending some of our girls to help. I found out about it this morning.' Her eyes probed deep into the heart of me. 'I've been selected. We leave tomorrow. I wasn't sure when I'd be back, so I wanted tonight to be special. I didn't know when I'd see you again.'

A man may die more than one death, I know, for this is what happened to me. I lost the power of hope. There were no words for what I wanted to say.

'We've had some good years, Harry. The best. Be thankful for that, I am.' Nan spoke so reasonably, but inside my body was breaking, separating into tiny splinters of flesh never to be whole again. I could not believe that any of this was happening. Our future had all been agreed upon.

'But we've always been true to each other, Nan. We were born for each other - how can we stop now? I need you. I love you.'

She forced a smile, the edges of her mouth creasing almost imperceptibly upwards.

'I know, Harry. I know. But maybe it's out of our control.' There was something in her voice, those eyes, which spoke of inner wisdom. Nan had seen this day approaching, a long, flat shadow haunting our own horizon.

'The thing to hate most in the world is a lie,' she continued, 'and we've never lived like that. We can't start now. It's good that we had our time together, but don't ask for more if this isn't possible.'

'I can't leave, Nan. I'll stay.' My words sounded puny. Impotent.

'Do what you must, Harry. Things might still work out. But remember darling, I will always love you.'

She leaned forwards to stroke my cheek and only now lost her composure. We stared into each other's eyes with no further words, as close as you can be to another person in that silence. It was a look that would have to last a lifetime.

My mind became flooded with thoughts of all the things we did and did not do. I remembered our first meeting, that tentative first kiss by the gunpost. I recalled the way she held out her arms for me to walk into her embrace, and the dance at the hospital. Our time at Dingli, night swimming. Gozo. I determined to study every detail of her face, so that I should never forget.

It was Nan who eventually spoke.

'Harry, will you please make love to me?'

She climbed above me, over me, and we gave ourselves completely on this, our last time. Until there was nothing left. When we kissed, I felt weightless. Cast adrift.

CHAPTER NINETEEN

I was completely numb inside, stumbling around in a daze. There was no way that I could return to barracks or stay near the hospital. Nan was leaving the next day, and I was being sent home. To be married, and have a child with Gwen. Everything about it was wrong. Unreal. Somehow, I discovered myself at Buskett Gardens, in the place where we had loved. It was here that tears climbed a ladder inside me, to finally break free.

We had always been in tune with each other, and I felt sure that Nan would come for me. She would find me like this, and make everything all right. I remembered the flicker of her eyelashes while she slept, the fullness of her lips. My mind touched slowly along the length of her body, of which I knew every detailed inch. When I reached the birthmark on her chest, a second wave of tears burst out and continued to fall. I reached for a prickly pear.

The needles popped one by one through the skin of my palm. Memories continued to snowball. There had been the enemy pilot at Dingli - he may as well have killed us if it should all now end like this. The canoe at Marsaxlokk - just once, I managed to stand, and Nan had tugged at my shorts to throw us both into the water. We had been so happy then. Fingers tightened about the fruit, a vague sensation of stickiness.

There was the dance at the hospital and, later, in the sea. But Gozo was the best. We had been safe, outside of time, and should never have returned. I glanced down at the hand that now formed a crimson fist, and still I felt nothing. There had been no sign of Nan to collect me. I remained in the gardens long after the sun had sunk out of the sky. The birds had stopped singing. I realised that I had cried outside, in public, without a care who should see me. Pain began to sing in my hand and my composure, as fragile as a seahorse, slowly began to return.

It was the middle of night when I returned to barracks, but I could not sleep. My thoughts refused to leave Nan. I remembered how she would touch people with her hands, always reassuring, to show how she cared. How I would lie encircling her, and she would bend forwards to allow our love. I pictured the home we should have set up together, a little villa in Xlendi, or maybe Fontana, on Gozo. Our first child, a boy. I was even thinking of names. I was filled with this great leftover love and it ate away at me, gnawing through my guts and breaking my heart.

The night was endless. At the first pale light of dawn, a whisper of birdsong, I understood that I had to see her again. I could not leave things as they were. I jumped out of bed, still in my clothes, grabbed shoes, and raced from the building.

It was dark outside my room, in constant shade from the barrack blocks. I ran across the courtyard and into the maze of M'tarfa, footsteps echoing loudly on the hard, unforgiving stone. I flung myself around and between the almond trees, heading as quickly as possible to the edge of town. I had to reach Nan in her quarters. Time was running out and so important.

Hammering on the solid wood of the door, I did not care who should hear me. Who should be woken from sweet, comfortable, dreaming. My hand hurt as it struck down repeatedly, and only then I remembered the prickly thorns of the pear. This pain felt good, proof of my intent, and I hit the wood with renewed strength. There was no reply heard from within.

My fingers reached instinctively for the handle. I pushed down and to my surprise the door clicked open. Maybe I wasn't too late, our relationship could still be salvaged, if only we had a plan.

I fell inside the room but she was not there. My eyes registered with dismay that her belongings had disappeared, the bed empty. I opened drawers in vain, ripped back the single sheet; not one trace of Nan remained. She had already left, on her way to Italy. I collapsed exhausted onto the bed, hopes crushed once again, staring at the white expanse of ceiling. The room still smelled of her perfume.

That day, the idea of work seemed impossible. I reported to Matron faking sickness, requesting an absence of twenty-four hours. There was nothing wrong with me physically, but the pain I experienced was real enough. Lack of sleep and the weight of worry I now carried must have been clearly evident, for Matron was very sympathetic. She told me not to return until I felt better. She knew that I was no shirker.

I walked to Mdina, past our field, and to Bastion Square. There was tightness in my chest making it a struggle just to breathe. I felt light-headed. The gunpost was now unmanned and there was nobody around to disturb the silence, but this meant nothing without Nan. I had become a man who cast no shadow, no reflection in any mirror. I stood alone under an angry sun and gazed out over the island.

The threads connecting us had been allowed a chance to snap, and for this I blamed only myself. I had been so determined not to make any mistakes this time, and should never have let her go so easily. Countless images swam in front of my eyes, teasing, chastising, before solidifying into a giant picture of her face. Those dark eyes, her hair, her smile. I was consumed with the awful realisation that you do not understand how to love someone properly until after they are gone.

The second day, I felt no better and did not return to work. There had been no further information regarding my own departure.

I walked to Buskett Gardens, thinking continuously of all the things I should have attempted to keep us together, and of all the things that might never now take place. The ground was stained where we once had lain, dark beads on the parched earth as if from a sudden shower. The light was dappled green above my head.

At Dingli Cliffs, our cove, resolve began to crystallise and take shape inside me. I sat on the narrow beach, shoes off, salt water washing over my feet. The sea was loud in my ears, and white birds floated high on the warm air. The islet of Filfa flickered on the horizon. Bright sunlight hurt my eyes; in four years on the island, I had never grown accustomed to this. I remembered all the times that we had come to this very spot, and my mind was then decided.

I was not going to leave. I would request to see the Colonel, to fight for my right to stay. If I could get the backing of Major Merryweather, I would argue that my experience was required in the hospital. If there should be a fresh outbreak of polio, or even typhoid, there was nobody else to replace me. To hell with any consequence. I would tell him the truth about Gwen, if he should let me. This still made no sense, because she had always stated her clear intention of never carrying another child. One was enough to bring into the world, after her own traumatic upbringing. I wondered as to her ulterior motives, for nothing was ever as it seemed with Gwen.

I would fight as hard as I could to remain on the island, whatever the punishment received. The only thing that I felt sure of was that I wanted to be with Nan. I'd never believed in anything as strongly. You could not and should not argue with fate, destiny, or nature, whatever you wanted to call it. We were right together, a couple; this was a simple, beautiful, truth.

The sea reached higher up my legs, and I began to rehearse the words of my defence. My case had to be strong, watertight, convincing. I had to show that my intentions were reasonable. I thought of the words I should say to Nan on her return, to make them perfect. Finally, I would get to meet her family. I could always convert to Catholicism, if necessary, for I did believe in a God. The sun began its descent from the sky, a ghostly shadow of myself cast into the darkening water.

It was the next day when the news arrived. Matron hurried into F Block, I had returned to work, and she asked me to join her outside. She tried but could not return my gaze.

I followed her into the gardens, past the fig tree, to stand at the low stone wall beyond the chapel. When she turned to face me, I noticed how pale and tired she looked, her face constricted with fresh worry. She reached out to take my hands before having a change of mind. Her arms dropped lifeless to her sides.

'Harold, there's something you must know.' She spoke so quietly, deliberately. She lowered her gaze to the ground. 'The boat to Bari was sunk, it hit a mine. There were no survivors, I'm so sorry.' She pressed my hands briefly between her own. 'If there's anything I can do to help, please tell me. I'll leave you alone now, but I really am sorry.'

She walked quickly towards the hospital, leaving me standing in silence. I couldn't believe it. It made no sense. Especially now, of all times, when the war was nearly won.

A brown bird landed in the pink oleander beside me, singing joyfully. A tiny lizard scuttled over my feet before darting nervously away. One giant red butterfly fluttered indolently about my head, and still I did not move. I could not move. Truth burnt a hole inside me and through me. I slowly understood how the greatest pain in life is when love moves in one direction only.

Nan was gone forever. Taken away from me. A memory. I thought about my prayers in the church at Ta Pinu, that I had believed to be acknowledged. My words, how only death could keep us apart. There had been the time on the cathedral steps in Gozo, when she had said she'd always love me. 'As long as I live.' Like the sea, she would never grow old.

An unspeakable loneliness rained down upon me, and how I wished we could have been married. That I had converted to Catholicism, to declare our love and make it real. I wished, too late, for a sign of permanence. I have no idea how long I stood. I cannot remember leaving the island.

Time seems to pass and the world keeps on turning. The night remains filled with newborn dreams. But after leaving Nan in her quarters, I never saw her again. From that moment, I was living someone else's life.

Author's Note

My father, Harold Edward Fisher, died in the Ramsay Ward of Buckland Hospital, Dover, on the twenty-eighth of October 1996. Known as Harry to his friends, he had worked here for over thirty years and died at the age of eighty-five. A charge nurse, this was his former ward. It fell on me, his only son, to carry out the heartbreaking task of sorting and clearing his possessions.

I discovered my father had indeed kept a lucky bear, given to him by one Dot Golding. There were books of old photographs, including some from Malta during the Second World War. I feel sure he would now be pleased that I keep his army medals, together with a letter from King George on receiving the British Empire Medal.

I also discovered notes relating to events that had occurred throughout his life. These were in no shape or form suitable for publication, and yet the story shone through to hold me captive. It would be a loss for this lifetime of history to be forgotten, and I determined that I would simply have to write it myself.

This I have done, making every effort to maintain the spirit of the original. In so doing, my father has returned from the dead.

Laurence Fisher, 2004.